Healing Wonders

Nature's Miracles Unveiled

To eat is a necessity, but to eat intelligently is an art.

— La Rochefoucauld

Healing Wonders
Nature's Miracles Unveiled

Dr. Rajat Trehan

Heal Your Body
New Delhi

Published by
Shhalaj Publishing House
Flat No. D-4, Landmark Apt., Plot 106-107
Vipin Garden, Dwarka Mod, New Delhi–110 059, India
Phone: +91-11-47529624; 8141882226
Email: support@shhalaj.com, ***Web:*** www.shhalaj.com

Printed in India

Cataloguing-in-Publication Data

Trehan, Rajat, 1971 – , author.
Healing Wonders: Nature's Miracles Unveiled / Dr. Rajat Trehan.

pages ; cm

Annotation: Practical guide on natural remedies and nutrition offering holistic approaches to common ailments, promoting sustainable wellness through lifestyle choices.

ISBN 13: 978-93-344-4075-1 (pbk) **ISBN 10:** 93-344-4075-9

1. Naturopathy. 2. Nutrition — Health aspects. 3. Alternative medicine. 4. Self-care, Health. 5. Holistic medicine.

LCC: RZ440 .T74 2025
DDC, 23rd ed.: 615.5 — Therapeutics, naturopathy & alternative medicine

Additional Entry:
Title: Nature's Miracles Unveiled

Dedication

Dedicated to the cherished memory of my dearly departed parents, the late P.J. Trehan and the late Jyoti Trehan.

In their enduring love, relentless dedication, and profound commitment, I find the guiding light that has shaped the person I am today.

May their legacy of love and resilience continue to inspire and guide me on life's journey

Disclaimer

About the author

Dr. Rajat Trehan, PhD, (Clinical Nutrition)

Dr. Rajat Trehan is a passionate advocate for holistic health and well-being. He empowers individuals to achieve optimal vitality through the transformative power of natural healing. Combining his extensive educational background, including a Ph.D. in Clinical Nutrition and a Master's in Nutritional Science, with over 20 years of experience, Dr. Trehan guides his clients on a journey towards optimal health.

Fueled by a mission to spread love, joy, and happiness through the power of plants, Dr. Trehan champions a unique approach focused on addressing the root causes of lifestyle diseases. He firmly believes in leveraging the synergy of dietary changes, natural therapies, and mindful lifestyle modifications to achieve holistic and sustainable results.

Beyond his clinical practice, Dr. Trehan is a dedicated thought leader, actively educating and empowering communities worldwide. He has touched the lives of thousands by successfully reversing chronic conditions like diabetes, arthritis, and liver disorders, offering a beacon of hope for those seeking natural solutions.

Dr. Trehan's infectious enthusiasm, deep scientific knowledge, and compassionate approach make him a trusted guide on your path to vibrant health. Through engaging lectures, workshops, and publications, he continues to inspire and empower individuals to embrace the transformative power of plant-based wellness.

Acknowledgement

Gratitude fills my heart as I sincerely thank the remarkable individuals whose steadfast support and expertise have played an indispensable role in the realisation of 'Healing Wonders: Nature's Miracles Unveiled.'

Mr. Rajan Dhir, your invaluable advice and insightful health discussion have been a guiding beacon. Our exploration of topics ranging from diet and nutrition to life's intricacies has truly enriched this book's essence. The 'agreeing to disagree' concept, exemplified through our discourse, embodies the spirit of nonjudgmental dialogue.

My brother, Dr. Rajeev Trehan, is an unwavering motivational source. He brings expertise in CVTS to Neotia Getwel Health Care Centre, Siliguri, and is a constant source of inspiration.

My sister-in-law, Dr. Meena Trehan, a Senior Consultant in Paediatric Cardiac Anaesthetist, is a steadfast pillar of support.

I extend immense gratitude to my colleagues for their invaluable support and assistance throughout this endeavour.

Mr. Parminder Singh Kakria and Mr. Karan Hari, mentors for life, have been unwavering motivators and inspirations on this profound journey.

My uncle, Mr. Sunil Badhwar, and Aunt Renu Badhwar deserve heartfelt thanks for their guidance and care while writing this book.

A special appreciation goes to Ankita Singh, my dedicated editor, who has been with me from the book's inception to completion. Your guidance and expertise have transformed my words into a polished work of art.

To my friends, your encouragement has been a driving force behind my work.

Lastly, heartfelt appreciation to Shhalaj Mittaal from Shhalaj Publishing House for the constant support, invaluable guidance, and seamless cooperation in bringing this book to a broader audience.

I sincerely thank the readers who have welcomed this book into their world. It has been a privilege to share this work with you, which was made possible by the remarkable individuals and entities mentioned above.

Warm regards,
Dr. Rajat Trehan

Preface

In Healing Wonders: Nature's Miracles Unveiled, I invite you to embark on a transformative and enlightening journey into the world of holistic well-being. Throughout this book, I, Dr. Rajat Trehan, a Clinical Nutritionist and Phytotherapist, explore the intricate tapestry that connects our body, mind, and spirit with the profound healing intelligence of nature. Each chapter serves as a gentle reminder that health is not merely the absence of disease but a dynamic state of balance—one that nature has always guided us toward.

This book delves deeply into the relationship between what we consume, what we avoid, and how these choices influence our vitality. Within these pages, you will find the essence of natural healing distilled into practical wisdom—remedies, insights, and reflections that illuminate the path to vibrant living. Drawing from years of experience in clinical nutrition and phytotherapy, I examine a wide spectrum of everyday conditions through an integrated and compassionate lens. Rather than merely describing symptoms and causes, I explore the underlying imbalances—nutritional, emotional, and environmental—that give rise to illness, and how mindful adjustments in our daily lives can restore harmony and health.

Healing Wonders is more than a book; it is a roadmap for rediscovering equilibrium in an increasingly fragmented world. Through its pages, you will uncover not just natural remedies but philosophies—ways of thinking and living that rekindle your connection with the Earth's rhythms. My aim is to empower you with knowledge that transcends prescriptions and quick fixes, encouraging you to become an active participant in your own healing journey. Each suggestion, formulation, and reflection is intended to help you listen deeply to your body and align your habits with the nurturing forces of nature.

Together, we will explore the timeless healing potential found in the simplest elements—air, sunlight, herbs, water, and food—and recognise that the most profound miracles often lie in the smallest acts of care. This book also emphasises prevention as the highest form of healing, inspiring readers to cultivate lifestyles that fortify both body and spirit.

As we journey through Healing Wonders: Nature's Miracles Unveiled, my purpose extends beyond sharing nutritional or therapeutic insights—it is to offer a framework for self-awareness and transformation. Healing, in its truest essence, begins with awareness and blossoms through alignment—with nature, with truth, and with oneself. By returning to the wisdom of the natural world, we discover not only solutions for disease but also pathways to peace, purpose, and resilience.

This book is, therefore, an invitation—a call to reconnect with the ancient yet ever-living wisdom of nature. It encourages you to view the world not as separate from yourself but as a living ally in your well-being. Join me in embracing a holistic approach to health that honours both scientific understanding and the healing intelligence of nature's bioactive compounds. Together, let us align ourselves with the rhythms of the Earth and unlock the miraculous potential that resides within and around us.

Introduction

Welcome to "Healing Wonders: Nature's Miracles Unveiled" by Dr. Rajat Trehan – your friendly guide to unravelling the secrets of well-being the natural way.

Have you ever wondered about the incredible connection between what we eat, the remedies nature provides, and our everyday health battles? Well, you're in for a treat! I'm Dr. Rajat Trehan, and I'm thrilled to take you on a journey exploring the wonders of holistic health.

In these pages, we'll discuss the things we munch on, the ones we should avoid, and the fantastic natural remedies just waiting to be discovered. There will be no jargon, just straightforward insights into common diseases we all encounter, sprinkled with a bit of wit and a whole lot of wisdom.

From symptoms to causes and even a bit of behind-the-scenes on our daily choices, we're diving into the nitty-gritty of what makes us tick (and sometimes, what makes us hiccup). Think of it as your go-to manual for decoding the language of your body and understanding the language of nature.

I'm not just here to drop knowledge bombs – I want this to be your go-to source for embracing a healthier and more balanced lifestyle. So, buckle up, grab a comfy seat, and let's navigate the fascinating world where health meets nature.

Here's to unlocking the "Healing Wonders: Nature's Miracles Unveiled" has tucked away just for you.

Contents

1

Acidity

Introduction

Do you often suffer from heartburn at night? Does your stomach feel bloated or gassy? Does your throat burn with juices and food backflowing from your gut? Well, it's a common situation encountered by nearly every individual across various age groups, known as acidity.

Acidity is characterised by the excessive production of acid in the stomach. This disruption not only leads to stomach discomfort but also gives rise to an array of symptoms, such as heartburn, regurgitation(the action of bringing swallowed food up again to the mouth), and abdominal pain. Understanding the triggers behind this heightened acid production is crucial in effectively managing and preventing its effects. As a pervasive ailment, exploring the multifaceted factors contributing to acidity can pave the way for improved healthcare strategies and enhanced well-being.

Causes

Some prevalent causes of acidity encompass:

Dietary Influences:

- Consumption of chillies, pepper, vinegar, and paprika-rich foods.
- Indulgence in deep-fried and oily foods.
- Excessive intake of caffeine from tea, coffee, and chocolate.
- Elevated consumption of table salt.
- A low-fibre diet.

- Overeating or erratic meal timings.
- Unwise practices such as reclining immediately after eating.
- Ingesting food right before intense physical exertion.

Lifestyle Elements:

- Frequent smoking habits.
- Excessive consumption of alcohol, carbonated drinks, or soda.
- Inadequate sleep duration.
- Lack of physical activity.

Medical Conditions and Medications:

- Heightened stress levels, anxiety, or depression.
- Stomach ailments include peptic ulcers, gastroesophageal reflux disease (GERD), and stomach cancer.
- The influence of certain medications like painkillers, antibiotics, chemotherapy drugs, and antidepressants.

Symptoms

The symptoms of acidity, also known as acid reflux or heartburn, can vary in intensity and presentation. Common symptoms include:

1. **Heartburn**: A burning sensation or discomfort in the chest, often behind the breastbone, that can intensify after meals or when lying down.

2. **Regurgitation**: A feeling of acid or food returning to the throat or mouth, sometimes accompanied by a sour or bitter taste.

3. **Chest Pain**: Some people may mistake acidity-related chest pain for a heart attack due to its similar location and sensation. It's important to differentiate between the two.

4. **Difficulty Swallowing**: A sensation of something stuck in the throat or difficulty swallowing food or liquids.

5. **Sore Throat**: Repeated exposure to stomach acid can irritate the throat, leading to a sore or scratchy throat.
6. **Cough**: Chronic coughing, especially at night or after meals, can be triggered by acid irritating the throat and airways.
7. **Hoarseness**: Acid reflux can lead to inflammation of the vocal cords, causing changes in voice quality or hoarseness.
8. **Feeling of a Lump**: A sensation of a lump or something being stuck in the throat (Globus sensation) can occur due to irritation from acid.
9. **Belching**: acidity may cause frequent belching or burping, as air swallowing accompanies acid.
10. **Nausea**: Some individuals with acid reflux may experience nausea or an uneasy feeling in the stomach.
11. **Bloating**: Excess stomach acid can disrupt the digestive process and cause excessive gas or bloating.

Foods to Avoid

To minimise acidity, one should avoid:

1. **Citrus Fruits**: Oranges, lemons, and grapefruits are highly acidic.
2. **Tomatoes**: Tomato-based products like sauces can trigger acidity.
3. **Spicy Foods**: Peppers and hot spices can irritate the stomach lining.
4. **High-Fat Foods**: Fried foods, fatty meats, and creamy dishes delay digestion.
5. **Chocolate**: Contains compounds that may relax the lower oesophageal sphincter.
6. **Caffeine**: Coffee, tea, and sodas can stimulate acid production.

7. **Carbonated Drinks:** Soda and fizzy beverages increase gas and pressure.
8. **Onions and Garlic:** Both can cause lower oesophageal sphincter relaxation.
9. **Mint:** Peppermint and spearmint can exacerbate symptoms.
10. **Alcohol:** Alcoholic beverages relax the LES(lower oesophageal sphincter) and boost acid production.
11. **Processed Foods:** Fast food and pre-packaged snacks are often high in fat and salt.

Foods to Eat

1. **Oatmeal:** Low in acidity and a soothing option for breakfast.
2. **Bananas:** Non-acidic and gentle on the stomach.
3. **Ginger:** Known for its anti-inflammatory properties.
4. **Leafy Greens:** Spinach, kale, and other greens are alkaline.
5. **Melons:** Watermelon and cantaloupe are less likely to trigger reflux.
6. **Lean Proteins:** Change to chicken, turkey, and fish rather than high-fat meats.
7. **Whole Grains:** Brown rice, whole wheat bread, and quinoa are kinder on digestion.
8. **Non-Citrus Fruits:** Apples, pears, and berries are less likely to cause acidity.
9. **Almonds:** Almonds can help neutralise stomach acid.
10. **Non-Caffeinated Herbal Teas:** Chamomile and liquorice root tea can ease discomfort.

Remedies

1. **Cold Milk:** Cold milk is a straightforward and effective home remedy for acidity. Its calcium content regulates excessive stomach acid production, absorbing acids and

providing relief. If you're not lactose-intolerant, cold milk is an excellent remedy, offering instant relief from stomach burning.

How to use: All it takes is a refreshing glass of cold milk.

2. **Ajwain**: Ajwain is a natural solution for abdominal discomfort, including indigestion and acid reflux. Its enzymes and thymol address gastric issues, providing relief.

How to use: Consume a pinch of ajwain with salt and chew it, or soak a tablespoon overnight in water and drink it the following day.

3. **Apple Cider Vinegar**: Apple cider vinegar, taken before meals, reduces acid reflux by balancing stomach pH levels by neutralising stomach acid, mainly as it's often linked to indigestion.

How to use: Blend 1 to 2 tablespoons of raw apple cider vinegar with a cup of water and consume this mixture once daily.

4. **Basil Leaves**: Tulsi (basil) is renowned as an excellent herb for various concerns, including acidity. Its soothing qualities swiftly alleviate the burning sensation and stomach acid formation.

How to use: Chew on a couple of leaves during the day, or if you like it, soak them in water and drink them regularly.

5. **Fennel seeds or saunf**: This solution alleviates acidity, heartburn, and related discomforts like bloating and stomach aches. You can have a mixture of saunf and mishri to help with digestion.

6. **Non-citrus fruits**: Bananas, apples, and melons (watermelon, honeydew, cantaloupe) are low-acid fruits, making them ideal for acid reflux. Their high fibre content aids in alleviating stomach discomfort.

7. **Coconut water**: Unsweetened coconut water, with its electrolytic properties, such as potassium, benefits acid reflux. It shifts the body's pH from acidic to basic, aiding in controlling reflux.
8. **Ginger**: Ginger's anti-inflammatory nature eases indigestion and heartburn by reducing stomach acid flow into the oesophagus and calming the stomach.

How to use: Experiment with incorporating ginger into different meals or infuse it in tea; alternatively, chew on a fresh ginger slice for relief.

References:

1. https://www.1mg.com/diseases/acidity-42?wpsrc=Google+Organic+Search
2. https://www.healthshots.com/healthy-eating/nutrition/8-foods-and-home-remedies-for-acidity/

2

Acne

Introduction

Don't eat chocolates, or else you will get acne. Don't eat oily food. It is terrible for your skin health, and you will surely get acne, if nothing else. You might have heard these kinds of statements almost every other day.

Acne is prevalent among teenagers, but that does not mean adults can never be prone to it. Anyone can experience acne at any stage of life. Everyone wants to look beautiful, but acne can sometimes make it challenging. It not only affects self-esteem but also contributes to emotional distress.

Acne occurs when a hair follicle gets plugged with oil or dead skin cells. It is a skin condition which can look like small red spots, blackheads, whiteheads, or pimples. Everyone tries to get smooth and clear skin, but dealing with acne can be emotionally challenging.

To overcome that emotional distress and lower self-esteem, read on to discover how to prevent acne.

Causes

What if I tell you that eating chocolate and oily food does not cause acne and is a myth? You will not believe me, right? Well, it is fitting that it is a myth. The factors that lead to acne differ from those that people usually think.

So, what are the factors that cause acne? Let's dive deep and find out.

There are four fundamental causes of acne:

1. Excessive production of oil (sebum)
2. Blocked hair follicles from oil and skin cells
3. Bacteria
4. Inflammation

The areas where acne appears commonly are your forehead, face, upper back, chest, and shoulders. These areas of our bodies are more prone to acne because most of the sebaceous (oil) glands are present there.

Symptoms

Symptoms of acne often manifest on the face and shoulders, but they can also be found on the chest, back, arms, legs, and buttocks. These skin changes may include:

1. Formation of crusts on skin bumps.
2. Development of cysts.
3. Presence of papules, which are small red bumps.
4. Formation of pustules, which are small red bumps containing white or yellow pus.
5. Redness surrounding the skin eruptions.
6. Potential scarring of the skin.
7. Presence of whiteheads.
8. Presence of blackheads.

Foods to Avoid

You might have heard people saying, don't eat that, don't eat this. Most of the time, we avoid eating anything sugary or oily when we have acne. However, knowing some of the specific things you should avoid eating if you have acne is important. Let's have a look at the foods that we should avoid eating.

1. **Refined Carbohydrates**: Be mindful of your intake of refined carbohydrates, as they may lead to increased blood sugar and insulin levels, potentially contributing to the development of acne. However, further research is necessary to establish a conclusive link.

2. **Dairy Products:** Exercise caution when consuming dairy products due to their association with greater acne severity. However, it remains uncertain whether a direct cause-and-effect relationship exists.
3. **Fast Food:** Consider reducing your fast food consumption, as it's been linked to a heightened risk of acne development. However, it's not entirely clear if fast food directly triggers acne.
4. **Chocolate:** Recent research suggests a possible connection between chocolate consumption and the development of acne. The exact reasons for this link and the strength of the relationship remain uncertain.
5. **Whey Protein Powder:** Limited data indicates a potential link between whey protein powder and the development of acne. More high-quality and up-to-date research is required to gain a better understanding of this association.

Remember that individual responses to these foods can vary, so it's crucial to monitor how your body reacts to different dietary choices and consult a healthcare professional if you have concerns about acne and your diet.

Foods to Eat

In contrast to the foods mentioned earlier that may contribute to acne, some alternative foods and nutrients can help maintain clear skin. These include:

1. **Omega-3 Fatty Acids:** Certain older studies have associated regularly consuming Omega-3s, known for their anti-inflammatory properties, with a reduced risk of acne.
2. **Probiotics:** Probiotics promote a healthy gut and balanced microbiome, reducing inflammation and the risk of acne development. Further research is needed to identify the most beneficial strains.
3. **Green Tea:** Green tea's polyphenols reduce inflammation and lower sebum production. Green tea extracts applied topically have been found to reduce acne severity.

4. **Turmeric**: Turmeric contains the anti-inflammatory polyphenol curcumin, which helps regulate blood sugar, improve insulin sensitivity, and inhibit acne-causing bacteria growth, potentially reducing acne.
5. **Vitamins A, D, E, and Zinc**: These nutrients play vital roles in skin and immune health and may help prevent acne.
6. **Paleolithic-Style Diets**: These diets, rich in lean meats, fruits, vegetables, and nuts and low in grains, dairy, and legumes, have been linked to lower insulin levels, which could benefit acne.
7. **Mediterranean-Style Diets**: A Mediterranean diet, abundant in fruits, vegetables, whole grains, legumes, fish, and olive oil, and low in dairy and saturated fats, has also been associated with reduced acne severity.

Remedies

Acne does harm your self-esteem, even though you don't see it happening. It happens slowly, and when it comes forward, you might feel anxious or depressed.

1. **Green Tea**: Antioxidants included in green tea help fight microorganisms and reduce inflammation.

How to use: It has been demonstrated that applying it to the skin dramatically reduces pimples.

2. **Essential Oils**: Certain essential oils, such as clove, cinnamon, rose, lavender, and rosemary, block microorganisms that cause acne.

How to use: Using these oils on the skin could lessen the appearance of blemishes or spots.

3. **Tea Tree Oil**: Tea tree oil combats germs that cause acne and irritation.

How to use: It has been demonstrated that applying it to the skin may sometimes lessen pimples.

4. **Aloe Vera**: Aloe vera gel can be applied topically to cure burns, mend wounds, and reduce inflammation.

How to use: Further research is necessary to determine its effectiveness when used alone, as it has demonstrated the ability to enhance the anti-acne effects of other treatments.

References:

1. https://www.pennmedicine.org/for-patients-and-visitors/patient-information/conditions-treated-a-to-z/acne
2. https://www.healthline.com/nutrition/foods-that-cause-acne#TOC_TITLE_HDR_7
3. https://www.healthline.com/nutrition/get-rid-of-pimples-fast#aloe-vera

3

Anaemia

Introduction

Anaemia is a prevalent medical condition in which red blood cells or the haemoglobin concentration within them is lower than normal. Haemoglobin is essential for oxygen transport, and when red blood cells are insufficient, abnormal, or lacking enough haemoglobin, blood's ability to deliver oxygen to body tissues diminishes. Hence, this deficiency reduces oxygen supply to body tissues, resulting in fatigue, weakness, and paleness.

Factors like inadequate iron intake, chronic diseases, or genetic disorders often cause it. Anaemia affects people of all ages. Its diverse forms include iron deficiency anaemia, the most common type globally. Other types stem from deficiencies in vitamin B12, folic acid, or chronic conditions such as kidney disease. However, addressing the underlying cause can treat it, and, in many cases, treatments include dietary adjustments or supplementation.

Causes

Certain types of Anaemia may be present from birth, while others can develop due to underlying chronic illnesses. Moreover, Various factors, including the following, can cause Anaemia:

1. **Nutrient Deficiencies**: Inadequate intake of nutrients like iron, vitamin B12, folate, and vitamin A can lead to Anaemia.

2. **Chronic Diseases:** Health issues like chronic kidney disease, inflammatory disorders, and certain cancers can interfere with red blood cell production and lead to Anaemia.
3. **Infections:** Diseases like malaria, HIV, tuberculosis, and parasitic infections can contribute to Anaemia by affecting red blood cell production or survival.
4. **Inherited Disorders:** Genetic conditions such as thalassaemia and sickle cell disease can cause abnormal red blood cells and lead to Anaemia.
5. **Gastrointestinal Disorders:** Conditions affecting the stomach and intestines can impact nutrient absorption, contributing to deficiencies that lead to Anaemia.
6. **Hormonal Factors:** Some hormonal disorders, like hypothyroidism, can influence red blood cell production and cause Anaemia.
7. **Pregnancy:** Increased blood volume can dilute red blood cells during pregnancy, leading to Anaemia.
8. **Medications:** Certain medications, such as chemotherapy drugs or those affecting the bone marrow, can disrupt red blood cell production.
9. **Blood Loss:** Acute or chronic bleeding from sources like ulcers, heavy menstrual periods, or trauma can result in Anaemia.
10. **Autoimmune Disorders:** Conditions like lupus or rheumatoid arthritis can lead to Anaemia by destroying red blood cells.
11. **Dietary Choices:** Vegetarian or vegan diets without proper planning might lack essential nutrients and contribute to Anaemia.

Symptoms

Anaemia can manifest with a range of symptoms, including:

1. **Fatigue:** Feeling unusually tired or weak, even with sufficient rest.
2. **Weakness:** Reduced physical strength and endurance.

3. **Paleness**: Skin and mucous membranes may appear pale due to decreased oxygen supply.
4. **Shortness of Breath**: Difficulty breathing, especially during exertion.
5. **Dizziness or Lightheadedness**: Feeling unsteady or faint.
6. **Headache**: Recurring or severe headaches can be a symptom.
7. **Cold Hands and Feet**: Reduced blood flow can cause extremities to feel cold.
8. **Rapid Heartbeat**: The heart might beat faster to compensate for oxygen deficiency.
9. **Cognitive Issues**: Difficulty concentrating and reduced cognitive function.
10. **Brittle Nails**: Nails might become brittle and break easily.
11. **Chest Pain**: Severe Anaemia can strain the heart, causing chest discomfort.
12. **Pale or Yellowish Skin**: Jaundice might occur if Anaemia is related to red blood cell destruction.
13. **Cravings for Non-Food Items**: Known as pica, this unusual craving might involve ice, dirt, or paper.

Recognising these symptoms and seeking medical evaluation can help diagnose and manage Anaemia appropriately.

Foods to Avoid

If you have Anaemia, it's essential to consider foods to avoid and foods to include in your diet to help manage the condition. Here are some foods that might be best limited or avoided:

1. **High Calcium Foods with Iron-Rich Meals**: Foods rich in calcium, like dairy products, can hinder iron absorption when consumed with iron-rich foods. It's advisable to avoid consuming these together.
2. **Caffeinated Beverages**: Coffee, tea, and certain soft drinks contain compounds that hinder iron absorption. Consuming them around meal times might impact iron intake. For example, according to a study cited in an

article, drinking a cup of coffee while eating a hamburger can reduce iron absorption by up to 39%. Drinking a cup of instant coffee with a piece of bread inhibits iron absorption by 60–90%.

3. **High-Fibre Foods with Iron Supplements**: Fibre-rich foods can reduce the absorption of non-heme iron (plant-based iron) found in supplements or vegetarian sources. You can space out consumption of these foods and iron supplements.
4. **Processed and Fast Foods**: These foods often lack important nutrients and can contribute to poor overall nutrition, particularly problematic for individuals with Anaemia.
5. **Excessive Alcohol**: Alcohol can impair the body's ability to absorb certain nutrients essential for managing Anaemia, such as vitamin B12 and folic acid.
6. **Certain Whole Grains**: While whole grains are generally nutritious, some contain compounds hindering iron absorption. Phytates in bran-containing grains can affect iron uptake.

It's important to note that moderation is vital. While avoiding the foods mentioned above, it's equally important to focus on a balanced diet rich in iron sources.

Foods to Eat

If you have Anaemia, including nutrient-rich foods in your diet can be beneficial. Focus on the following:

1. **Iron-rich foods**: Include sources of heme iron (found in animal products) like lean meats, poultry, and seafood. Non-heme iron (plant-based) sources include beans, lentils, tofu, spinach, and fortified cereals.
2. **Vitamin B12 Foods**: Consume animal products like meat, fish, eggs, and dairy, or choose fortified plant-based options like fortified cereals and plant-based milk alternatives.

3. **Folate-Rich Foods**: Folic acid, also called folate in its natural state, belongs to the B-group vitamins and serves various crucial roles. For instance, it collaborates with vitamin B12 to create healthy red blood cells. So, including leafy greens, beans, lentils, asparagus, and fortified grains can boost folate intake.
4. **Vitamin C-rich foods**: Vitamin C enhances non-heme iron absorption. Opt for citrus fruits, berries, bell peppers, broccoli, and tomatoes.
5. **Lean Proteins**: Incorporate lean proteins like poultry, fish, and legumes, which provide essential amino acids for red blood cell production.
6. **Nuts and Seeds**: Snack on nuts and seeds, such as almonds, pumpkin seeds, and sunflower seeds, to get a mix of nutrients, including iron and healthy fats.
7. **Whole Grains**: Choose fortified whole grains like brown rice and quinoa to ensure a balanced intake of nutrients.
8. **Leafy Greens**: Dark leafy greens, such as spinach and kale, contain a combination of iron and other essential nutrients.
9. **Eggs**: Eggs provide iron, vitamin B12, and protein, making them a valuable addition to an anaemia-friendly diet.
10. **Dried Fruits**: Snacking on dried fruits like raisins, apricots, and prunes offers iron and other nutrients.
11. **Liver (in moderation)**: The liver is a rich source of heme-iron and B vitamins, but due to its high vitamin A content, it's important to avoid overconsuming it.

Remember to maintain a balanced diet and consider any dietary restrictions you may have. Consulting a healthcare professional can help you tailor your diet to manage Anaemia effectively.

Remedies

1. **Beetroot**: This vegetable can fully help cure your Anaemia due to its natural iron content. Beetroot aids in elevating haemoglobin levels in the blood, leading to improved oxygen levels over time.

   How to use: You can enjoy beetroot cooked as a raw salad or freshly blended beetroot juice.

2. **Moringa Leaves**: Abundant in iron, vitamins A, C, and magnesium, moringa leaves are a remarkable source of nutrition. With 28 mg of iron per serving, they surpass spinach. Incorporating moringa leaves into your diet is recognised as enhancing haemoglobin and red blood cell counts.

   How to use: To prepare, finely chop 20-25 moringa leaves, create a paste, and mix with a teaspoon of jaggery powder. Consume this mixture during breakfast to boost your iron levels effectively.

3. **Sesame seeds**: Abundant in nutrients like iron, copper, zinc, selenium, and vitamins B6, E, and folate, sesame seeds offer substantial benefits. Regularly consuming black sesame seeds enhances haemoglobin levels and facilitates iron absorption.

   How to use: To prepare, dry roast one tablespoon of black sesame seeds, combine them with a teaspoon of honey and shape them into a ball. Regularly enjoy this nutritious ladoo to elevate your iron levels effectively.

These remedies, along with the foods listed in the 'foods to eat' section, can significantly help manage anaemia.

Remember, if you suspect you have Anemia, it's important to consult a healthcare provider for proper diagnosis and treatment. These home remedies should be considered complementary to medical advice and not a substitute for professional medical care.

References:

1. https://my.clevelandclinic.org/health/diseases/3929-anemia
2. https://www.who.int/health-topics/anaemia#tab=tab_1
3. https://www.vinmec.com/en/pharmaceutical-information/use-medicines-safely/do-coffee-and-caffeine-inhibit-iron-absorption/#:~:text=Some%20studies%20have%20shown%20coffee,absorption%20by%2060%E2%80%9390%25.
4. https://www.haiderian.co.uk/info.aspx?p=15#:~:text=Folic%20acid%20has%20several%20important,form%20healthy%20red%20blood%20cells
5. https://pharmeasy.in/blog/home-remedies-for-anaemia/
6. https://www.netmeds.com/health-library/post/anemia-5-awesome-natural-remedies-to-boost-your-iron-levels

4

Anorexia Nervosa

Introduction

Anorexia nervosa is a serious eating disorder and psychological implications characterised by a distorted body image and an intense fear of gaining weight, leading to self-imposed starvation and extreme weight loss. Individuals with anorexia often perceive themselves as overweight, regardless of actual body size.

This mental health condition affects both physical and psychological well-being, causing serious health complications such as nutritional deficiencies, organ damage, and even death.

Typical behaviours include restricted food intake, excessive exercise, and obsession with calorie counting. Anorexia predominantly affects adolescents and young adults, and early intervention is crucial for effective treatment and recovery.

Causes

1. **Biological**: genes, hormones, brain chemicals
2. **Environmental**: pressure to be thin, unrealistic body images
3. **Psychological**: negative body image, perfectionism, OCD

Symptoms

Individuals grappling with anorexia nervosa exhibit weight loss and uphold their meagre weight through various means. While some impose strict limits on their calorie intake, others exercise excessively. Specific individuals resort to a binge-and-purge approach akin to those with bulimia, and some rely on laxatives, vomiting, or diuretics to eliminate calories. If you are dealing with anorexia nervosa, you may experience the following symptoms:

1. Inability to maintain a healthy weight
2. Persistent fatigue
3. Insomnia
4. Skin exhibiting a yellow or blotchy appearance and being covered with soft, fine hairs
5. Thinning or loss of hair
6. Constipation
7. Absence of menstruation for more than three cycles
8. Dry skin
9. Low blood pressure

Furthermore, you might observe certain behaviours such as:

1. Excessive exercise
2. Manipulating food on the plate rather than consuming it or cutting food into small pieces
3. Irritability
4. Withdrawal from social activities
5. A prevailing sense of depression
6. Denial of hunger
7. Use of diuretics, laxatives, or diet pills

Foods to Avoid

1. **Processed foods:** These foods are full of calories but don't have many nutrients. They can make you feel tired and sluggish, and they can also lead to weight gain.

2. **Sugary drinks:** These drinks are also full of calories and don't have many nutrients. They can make you feel jittery and can also lead to weight gain.

3. **Alcoholic beverages:** Alcohol can upset your stomach and make you throw up. It can also make you feel dehydrated, which can make your anorexia worse.

4. **Aerated drinks**: These drinks are full of calories and lack nutrients. They can also make you feel bloated and lead to weight gain.
5. **Refined flour**: This type of flour is processed and doesn't have much fibre, making you feel constipated and lead to blood sugar spikes.
6. **Spicy Food**: These foods can irritate your stomach and make you throw up. They can also make your heartburn worse.
7. **Saturated and trans fats**: These fats are hard to digest and can make you feel sick. They can also raise your cholesterol levels and increase your risk of heart disease.
8. **Teas and coffees**: These drinks can make you feel restless and anxious. They can also make you throw up.
9. **Canned and preserved foods**: These foods are often processed and have lost many nutrients. They can also be high in sodium and preservatives, which can make you feel bloated and uncomfortable.

Foods to Eat

Fruits and vegetables are an important part of a healthy diet for everyone, including people with anorexia. Most fruits and vegetables are safe to eat, but some people may have trouble digesting certain types, such as apples or carrots. Talk to your doctor or nutritionist to determine which fruits and vegetables are best for you.

Protein is also crucial for people with anorexia. Lean proteins like chicken, fish, tofu, and beans are good choices. However, people with kidney problems may need to limit their protein intake. Talk to your doctor or nutritionist to determine how much protein suits you.

Whole grains are a healthy carbohydrate that people with anorexia can eat. They provide energy and essential vitamins and minerals. However, people with digestive problems may need to avoid whole grains. Talk to your doctor or nutritionist to determine if whole grains suit you.

Dairy products are a good source of calcium and other nutrients and are generally safe for people with anorexia. However, people with lactose intolerance may need to avoid dairy products. Talk to your doctor or nutritionist to find out if dairy products are right for you.

Remedies

1. **Lemon-Mint Honey Water**: This is a refreshing and nutritious drink. You can add a pinch of salt and cumin seed powder to taste. Vitamin C is a powerful antioxidant that can help protect your cells from damage.
2. **Ajwain (carom seeds)**: Take one teaspoon of Ajwain with water three times a day to help increase your appetite.
3. **Hing (asafoetida)**: To help improve your appetite, take a pinch of hing with 1 teaspoon of pure bilona cow ghee (grass-fed cow) before meals.
4. **Pineapple**: Pineapple can help increase your appetite.
5. **Papaya**: Papaya can help restore your appetite.

Recommendations

1. Chew your food slowly and thoroughly to increase meal satisfaction and decrease consumption.
2. Start with smaller portions and gradually adjust as you become more comfortable.
3. Avoid eating late at night to improve sleep quality and prevent weight gain.
4. Consult with a nutritionist or healthcare professional to devise a meal plan tailored to your needs.

5. If experiencing depression or other psychological issues, consider seeking assistance from a psychological therapist to develop coping strategies and manage symptoms effectively.

Resources:

1. https://www.mayoclinic.org/diseases-conditions/anorexia-nervosa/symptoms-causes/syc-20353591
2. https://www.healthline.com/health/anorexia-nervosa#causesn-levels

5

Arthritis

Introduction

You may have heard of arthritis or know someone who suffers from it. This condition directly affects the joints and involves both inflammation and degeneration. Arthritis is most commonly found in the feet, hands, lower back, hips, and knees.

Arthritis is not a single disease but rather a term referring to more than a hundred different types and related conditions. It affects people of all ages, sexes, and races. Although it is often associated with older adults, it can also occur in younger individuals. Women are more likely to develop arthritis than men.

Types of Arthritis

Several common types of arthritis include:

1. **Osteoarthritis:** Often referred to as "wear-and-tear" arthritis, this condition results from repeated stress that causes joint cartilage to break down. It is the most common form of arthritis.
2. **Ankylosing Spondylitis:** A type of arthritis that primarily affects the spine, particularly the lower back.
3. **Juvenile Arthritis (JA):** A condition in which the immune system attacks tissues surrounding the joints. It typically affects children aged sixteen or younger.

4. **Gout:** A disorder caused by the accumulation of uric acid crystals in the joints.
5. **Psoriatic Arthritis:** Inflammation of the joints that occurs in some people with psoriasis, a chronic autoimmune skin condition.
6. **Rheumatoid Arthritis (RA):** A condition in which the immune system attacks the synovial membranes that line the joints.

Causes

The causes of arthritis vary depending on the type. Contributing factors may include:

1. **Injury**, which can lead to degenerative arthritis.
2. **Abnormal metabolism**, resulting in conditions such as gout and calcium pyrophosphate deposition disease (CPPD).
3. **Genetic predisposition**, particularly in cases of osteoarthritis.
4. **Infections**, such as Lyme disease, which can trigger arthritis symptoms.
5. **Immune system dysfunction**, as seen in rheumatoid arthritis and lupus.

Most types of arthritis are influenced by multiple factors. Some forms arise without an apparent cause and may seem to occur unpredictably.

Symptoms

Symptoms of arthritis vary depending on the type and may:

1. Develop gradually or appear suddenly.
2. Come and go or persist over time.

COMMON WARNING SIGNS INCLUDE:

1. Joint pain
2. Swelling
3. Stiffness
4. Difficulty moving a joint

Some forms of arthritis may also present unique symptoms:

1. Juvenile RA can lead to eye problems.
2. Septic arthritis can cause fever and severe joint pain.

Foods To Avoid

Certain foods may exacerbate arthritis symptoms. It is advisable to:

1. **Limit sugar**: Excess sugar can worsen inflammation.
2. **Avoid processed foods**: These often contain trans fats, which raise bad cholesterol and lower good cholesterol.
3. **Reduce gluten**: For some individuals, gluten may trigger flare-ups.
4. **Processed foods:** Highly processed foods can elevate blood sugar, leading to increased inflammation.
5. **Quit smoking and reduce alcohol consumption**: Both can contribute to inflammation.
6. **Trans fats**: Found in fried foods, some dairy products, beef, and certain vegetable oils. These fats elevate bad cholesterol levels and reduce good cholesterol, worsening arthritis symptoms.
7. **Cut back on salt**: Excess sodium can lead to water retention and joint stiffness.
8. **Limit advanced glycation end products (AGEs)**: These compounds, produced by cooking at high temperatures or prolonged storage, can increase inflammation.

Following these dietary tips can help reduce inflammation and better manage arthritis symptoms.

Foods to Eat

Incorporating the following foods into your diet may help prevent pain and reduce joint inflammation:

1. Turmeric
2. Water
3. Mushroom
4. Omega-3 fatty acids
5. Organosulfur compounds
6. Dark green leafy vegetables
7. Nuts
8. Cruciferous vegetables

These foods can support joint health and decrease stiffness.

Remedies

1. **Water**: Essential for overall health and for flushing toxins from the body. Staying hydrated helps reduce inflammation and ease joint pain.
2. **Ginger**: Known for its anti-inflammatory properties, ginger helps manage pain and stiffness.
3. **Omega-3 fatty acids**: Found in flaxseeds, walnuts, and fish, these are vital for reducing inflammation and improving cardiovascular, eye, and joint health.
4. **Green tea**: Contains epigallocatechin gallate (EGCG), a potent anti-inflammatory compound beneficial for arthritis and inflammatory bowel conditions.
5. **Nuts**: Generate body heat, making them especially helpful for joint pain in colder months. They also support cardiovascular and musculoskeletal health.

6. **Organosulfur compounds**: Present in garlic, onions, and cruciferous vegetables; these compounds reduce inflammatory enzyme activity.
7. **Dark green leafy vegetables**: Rich in antioxidants, they help lower inflammation levels in individuals with arthritis.

Resources:

"Arthritis is Reversible: A Strategic Approach" by Dr. Rajat Trehan

6

Asthma

Introduction

Have you ever experienced a whistling sound while exhaling or felt short of breath? These symptoms often occur when your airways narrow and swell, leading to increased mucus production—a condition known as asthma.

Although asthma is considered not fully curable but managable, individuals can manage and potentially reverse its symptoms. Phytotherapy offers some hope in this regard. Because asthma symptoms frequently change over time, it is essential for you and your healthcare provider to monitor them and adjust treatments as needed.

Causes

Let's explore the causes of asthma.

1. **Family History**: Having a parent with asthma increases the risk three- to sixfold.
2. **Allergies:** A family history of allergies raises the likelihood of developing asthma.
3. **Viral Respiratory Infections:** Childhood wheezing caused by viral infections may lead to chronic asthma.
4. **Occupational Exposures:** Workplace elements such as dust, chemical fumes, and mould can induce asthma.
5. **Smoking**: Cigarette smoke, including maternal smoking during pregnancy, elevates asthma risk.

6. **Air Pollution:** Exposure to ozone and other pollutants in smog increases the likelihood of asthma.
7. **Obesity:** Overweight individuals, including children and adults, face a higher risk of asthma due to low-grade inflammation.

Poverty and limited health awareness often result in greater exposure to allergens and delayed medical care, increasing the risk of developing conditions like asthma and other allergies, or worsening their symptoms.

Symptoms

Asthma symptoms differ widely from person to person. For some, they occur only occasionally; for others, they may be triggered by specific factors such as physical activity, cold air, or emotional stress. In more severe cases, symptoms can be persistent and interfere with daily life. One common type, allergy-induced asthma, is triggered by airborne allergens such as pollen, mould spores, cockroach droppings, or pet dander.

Common signs and symptoms include:

1. Shortness of breath
2. Chest tightness or pain
3. Wheezing during exhalation, especially in children
4. Sleep disturbances caused by breathlessness, coughing, or wheezing
5. Coughing or wheezing exacerbated by respiratory infections such as the cold or flu

Indicators of worsening asthma include:

1. More frequent or bothersome symptoms
2. Increased difficulty breathing, as measured by a peak flow meter
3. More frequent use of quick-relief inhalers

Situational triggers may include:

1. Exercise-induced asthma, often worsened by cold, dry air
2. Occupational asthma, triggered by workplace irritants such as chemical fumes or dust

Foods to Avoid

Certain foods may trigger asthma symptoms. Always consult a healthcare provider before making major dietary changes.

1. **Sulfites:** Sulfites, a type of preservative, can worsen asthma. They are found in wine, dried fruits, pickled foods, maraschino cherries, shrimp, and bottled lemon or lime juice.
2. **Gas-Inducing Foods:** Large meals or gas-producing foods can press against the diaphragm, especially in individuals with acid reflux, leading to chest tightness and asthma flares. Examples include beans, cabbage, carbonated drinks, onions, garlic, and fried foods.
3. **Salicylates:** Rarely, some people with asthma are sensitive to salicylates—natural compounds found in coffee, tea, and certain herbs and spices.
4. **Artificial Ingredients:** Processed and fast foods often contain preservatives, flavorings, and colorings that may trigger asthma symptoms in sensitive individuals.
5. **Common Allergens:** Asthma sufferers with food allergies may react to dairy products, shellfish, wheat, or tree nuts. Identifying and avoiding these allergens can improve symptom management.

Foods to Eat

There is no specific diet for asthma, but certain nutrients may support lung function.

1. **Vitamin D:** Adequate intake may reduce asthma attacks in children aged 6 to 15. Sources include salmon, fortified milk and orange juice, and eggs. If you are allergic to milk or eggs, avoid them, as they may provoke symptoms.
2. **Vitamin A:** A 2018 study found lower vitamin A levels in children with asthma. Higher levels were associated with improved lung function. Sources include carrots, cantaloupe, sweet potatoes, and leafy greens such as romaine lettuce, kale and spinach.
3. **Apples:** Research published in Nutrition Journal suggests regular apple consumption is linked to a lower risk of asthma and improved lung function.
4. **Bananas:** A study in the European Respiratory Journal found that bananas may reduce wheezing in asthmatic children, likely due to their antioxidant and potassium content.
5. **Magnesium:** Low magnesium levels in children aged 11 to 19 have been linked to reduced lung function. Foods high in magnesium include spinach, pumpkin seeds, Swiss chard, dark chocolate, and salmon.

Remedies and their usage

1. **Garlic**

- Add fresh garlic to meals for its anti-inflammatory benefits.
- Use it in salads, soups, or sauces.
- Though conclusive evidence is lacking, garlic may help alleviate symptoms.

2. **Ginger**

- Brew ginger tea by steeping fresh slices in hot water.
- Incorporate grated ginger into recipes or smoothies.
- Ginger may help manage severe asthma symptoms.

3. **Honey**

- Mix honey into herbal teas.
- Combine with other ingredients such as cumin, as noted in a 2019 study.
- Always consult a healthcare provider before using honey therapeutically.

4. Omega-3 Oils

- Consume fatty fish such as salmon or mackerel.
- Add flaxseeds to smoothies, yogurt, or salads.
- If you're taking high-dose oral steroids, check with your doctor before increasing omega-3 intake, as interactions may occur.

Resources:

1. https://www.mayoclinic.org/diseases-conditions/asthma/symptoms-causes/syc-20369653
2. https://www.lung.org/lung-health-diseases/lung-disease-lookup/asthma/learn-about-asthma/what-causes-asthma
3. https://www.healthline.com/health/asthma/asthma-diet#foods-to-eat
4. https://www.healthline.com/health/severe-asthma/natural-remedies#food

7

Backache

Introduction

Most people experience backache at some point in their lives. While it is generally not a serious concern for those under the age of 60, it remains one of the leading reasons individuals seek medical attention and miss work.

Fortunately, backache can often be managed at home through minor lifestyle adjustments. A sedentary lifestyle is a common culprit. In many cases, back pain resolves within a few weeks with self-care. Before we discuss prevention, let us first explore the possible causes.

Causes

Back pain frequently occurs without a clearly identifiable cause detectable by diagnostic tests or imaging. However, common associated conditions include:

1. **Muscle or Ligament Strain:** Repeated heavy lifting or sudden awkward movements can strain back muscles and spinal ligaments, particularly in individuals with poor physical conditioning. This strain may result in painful spasms.
2. **Bulging or Ruptured Discs:** Discs act as cushions between the vertebrae. When they bulge or rupture, they may press on nearby nerves. However, such disc issues do not always cause pain and are sometimes incidentally discovered during imaging for other reasons.

3. **Arthritis:** Osteoarthritis can affect the lower back and may lead to spinal stenosis, a narrowing of the space around the spinal cord.
4. **Osteoporosis:** Brittle, porous bones in the spine may fracture easily, resulting in significant pain.
5. **Ankylosing Spondylitis (Axial Spondyloarthritis):** This inflammatory condition can cause some spinal bones to fuse, reducing the spine's flexibility.

Symptoms

1. **Diverse Pain Patterns:** Back pain may present as localised discomfort or as a widespread sensation across the back. It may also radiate to the buttocks, legs, or abdomen.
2. **Variable Intensity:** Pain severity varies between individuals. It may worsen with lifting, bending, resting, sitting, or standing for extended periods.
3. **Dynamic Nature:** Back pain often comes and goes. Morning stiffness is common but typically improves with movement.
4. **Associated Symptoms:** Pain may radiate to the buttocks, hips, or legs, and may be accompanied by numbness or weakness in the lower extremities.
5. **Red Flags for Medical Attention:** Seek medical advice if:
    - The pain persists beyond a few weeks.
    - The pain is accompanied by numbness or tingling, severe, unrelieved pain, a recent fall or injury, urinary incontinence, leg weakness, fever, or unexplained weight loss.

Foods to Avoid

1. **Sugary Foods:** These can contribute to inflammation and weight gain, exacerbating back pain. Artificial sweeteners may have similar effects.

2. **Vegetable Oil**: While omega-6 fatty acids are essential in moderation, excess intake may promote inflammation. Opt for olive oil, which contains healthier monounsaturated fats.
3. **Refined Grains**: Refined carbohydrates—found in foods such as white bread, cereal, and pizza—can spike insulin levels and promote inflammation. Choose whole grains instead.
4. **Dairy Products**: Although often recommended for bone health, dairy can be inflammatory for some individuals, especially those who have difficulty digesting it.
5. **Processed Corn Products**: These can increase insulin levels and trigger inflammation. Unprocessed corn is a better alternative.
6. **Red Meat**: While a source of protein, red meat contains Neu5Gc, a compound that may contribute to inflammation. Limiting intake may help alleviate symptoms.
7. **Chemically Processed Foods**: Avoid foods with artificial additives, colorings, and preservatives. These chemicals can trigger inflammation—always read labels carefully.

Foods to Eat

Vitamin D enhances calcium absorption and is essential for bone health, particularly in the vertebrae. Consult your physician to determine whether you need a supplement.

1. **Calcium-Rich Foods**: Sources include spinach, kale, collards, and sardines. A calcium-rich diet helps maintain strong bones.
2. **Vitamin D-Rich Foods**: Natural sources include tuna, salmon, mushrooms, cheese, and egg yolks.

Remedies

1. Cold and Heat Therapy

- **Immediately After Injury:** Apply a cold compress or ice pack to numb the area and reduce swelling.
- **After 48 Hours:** Switch to heat therapy using a heating pad or hot water bottle to relax muscles and improve blood flow.
- **Note:** Heat is most effective during the first week.

2. Limited Bed Rest

While bed rest was once commonly prescribed, it is now recommended only briefly, if pain prevents movement. Extended rest can lead to stiffness and worsen symptoms.

3. Physical Activity

Regular exercise builds strength and flexibility, reducing the likelihood of future injury and supporting healing. A well-rounded program—ideally designed with input from a healthcare professional—should include:

- Aerobic exercises
- Strength training
- Flexibility exercises

4. Complementary Therapies

These therapies may be used in conjunction with conventional care:

- **Acupuncture:** Uses fine needles to stimulate specific points.
- **Spinal Manipulation:** Chiropractors apply pressure to align the spine.
- **Therapeutic Massage:** Helps relax sore muscles.
- **Movement-Based Therapies:** Practices such as yoga and tai chi strengthen and stretch the back.

- **Effectiveness:** While results vary, these therapies often work best as part of a comprehensive treatment plan.

NOTE: For more details, read "Arthritis is Reversible" by Dr. Rajat Trehan

References:

1. https://www.mayoclinic.org/diseases-conditions/back-pain/symptoms-causes/syc-20369906
2. https://www.goodpath.com/learn/is-an-anti-inflammatory-diet-good-for-back-pain/
3. https://www.niams.nih.gov/health-topics/back-pain
4. https://www.texasspineclinic.com/foods-to-avoid-while-experiencing-back-pain/
5. https://www.health.harvard.edu/pain/home-remedies-for-low-back-pain

8

Boils

Introduction

A boil is a painful, pus-filled bump that forms under the skin when bacteria infect and inflame a hair follicle. Boils usually begin as red or purple tender nodules, gradually enlarging and becoming more painful as pus accumulates. Eventually, the boil bursts and drains.

Boils most commonly occur on the face, the back of the neck, armpits, thighs, and buttocks. While a single boil can typically be treated at home, avoid poking or squeezing it, as doing so may spread the infection.

Causes

- **Bacterial Infection**: Most boils are caused by Staphylococcus aureus, a bacterium commonly found on the skin or in the nose.
- **Pus Buildup**: A boil forms when pus accumulates beneath the skin's surface.
- **Entry Points**: Breaks in the skin—such as cuts, insect bites, or abrasions—can allow bacteria to enter and trigger infection.

Risk Factors

Several factors can increase the risk of developing boils:

- **Close Contact**: Living with or being in close physical contact with someone who has a staph infection, especially a boil or carbuncle, raises the risk.

- **Diabetes:** High blood sugar levels can impair the body's ability to fight skin infections.
- **Skin Conditions:** Conditions such as acne and eczema compromise the skin's barrier and increase vulnerability to infections.
- **Weakened Immunity:** A compromised immune system reduces the body's ability to resist bacterial infections, making one more prone to boils and carbuncles.

Symptoms

Boils may appear anywhere on the skin but are especially common in areas with hair and prone to friction or sweating, such as the face, neck, armpits, thighs, and buttocks.

Common signs and symptoms include:

- A painful, red bump that may grow to more than 2 inches (5 cm) in diameter
- Surrounding skin that becomes red or purple and swollen
- Gradual enlargement of the bump as it fills with pus
- Development of a yellow or white tip that eventually ruptures and drains

Foods to Avoid

1. Reduce consumption of hot and dry foods (e.g., eggs, chickpeas, onions, and chili), as well as hot and moist foods (e.g., sugar, white flour products, cheese, and mutton).
2. Avoid heavily spiced and fried foods, as well as refined and sugary options.
3. For a balanced diet, steer clear of cashew nuts, pecans, peanuts, eggs, cheese, pickles, processed meats, and chocolate.

Foods to Eat

1. Prioritise cold and moist foods such as carrots, cucumbers, lettuce, and rice. Follow with cold and dry options like citrus fruits, yogurt, fish, and beans.
2. Drink at least three liters of water daily.
3. Choose a high-fibre diet rich in fruits and vegetables to support regular bowel movements.
4. Incorporate raw or lightly steamed vegetables and fresh fruits into your meals.
5. Consider a monthly cleansing fast to help eliminate accumulated toxins from the body under the guidance of a healthcare provider.
6. Replace milky tea or coffee with rooibos tea and lemon juice for a healthier beverage option.

Herbal and Home Remedies

- Apply a warm compress to the affected area to help the boil come to a head and promote natural drainage.
- Cover the boil with a soft cloth pouch containing a slice of onion or tomato, a crushed garlic clove, or a used, cooled tea bag for additional relief.

References

- Mayo Clinic. "Boils and Carbuncles." https://www.mayoclinic.org/diseases-conditions/boils-and-carbuncles/symptoms-causes/syc-20353770
- Tibb Health Sciences. "Boils." https://www.tibb.co.za/ailments/boils.pdf

9

Common Cold

Introduction

Aaachhoouuu!!

"God bless you!"

You've likely heard this in your home, school, public places, or workplace—it's a sign someone has caught a cold.

The common cold, caused by viruses, affects the nose and throat. Although generally harmless, it can be quite uncomfortable. Adults may experience two or three colds per year, while infants and young children tend to get them more frequently. Recovery typically takes seven to ten days, though symptoms may last longer in smokers. Medical care is usually unnecessary unless symptoms persist or worsen.

Causes

Several viruses can cause the common cold, with **rhinoviruses** being the most prevalent.

A cold virus typically enters the body through the **mouth, eyes, or nose** and spreads via:

- Airborne droplets when someone coughs, sneezes, or speaks
- Direct contact with someone who has a cold
- Sharing items like dishes, towels, toys, or phones
- Touching your eyes, nose, or mouth after contact with the virus

Risk factors include:

- Close contact with individuals who have a cold
- Seasonal influence (more common in fall and winter, though possible year-round)
- Age (infants and young children are more susceptible than adults)

Symptoms

Cold symptoms usually appear **one to three days** after exposure to a virus.

Common symptoms include:

- Runny or stuffy nose
- Sore or scratchy throat
- Cough
- Sneezing
- General feeling of unwellness
- Mild body aches or headache
- Low-grade fever

Mucus may begin clear and become thicker, yellow, or green—this colour change is normal and indicates the body is fighting the infection.

Peak symptoms typically occur within **two to three days** and may include:

- Sneezing
- Nasal congestion or discharge
- Sore throat
- Cough
- Postnasal drip
- Watery eyes
- Fever (not always present)

Symptoms such as nasal congestion and cough may **persist for 10 to 14 days** but usually improve gradually.

Foods to Avoid

To support your immune system, avoid foods that promote inflammation or weaken your defences:

- Foods high in added sugar (e.g., desserts, cookies, ice cream, sweetened soft drinks)
- Highly processed foods (e.g., packaged snacks, frozen dinners, fast food)
- Alcohol and caffeinated beverages (e.g., energy drinks), which can dehydrate and stress your system

Such foods can hinder recovery by exacerbating inflammation and impairing immune response.

Foods to Eat

Though no food can cure a cold, several can help strengthen your immune system and boost energy. Try incorporating these into light meals or snacks:

- **Chicken soup**: A time-tested remedy that soothes the throat, provides hydration, and eases nasal congestion.
- **Yogurt with fruit**: Rich in probiotics to support immunity. Choose plain Greek yogurt for added protein; sweeten naturally with honey, which has antiviral properties.
- **Avocado toast**: Avocados offer healthy fats that reduce inflammation. Use whole-grain bread for extra nutrients.
- **Oatmeal**: Provides energy, fibre, and beta-glucan, which may benefit immune health.

Remedies

- **Stay hydrated**: Drink water, clear broths, juice, or warm lemon water. Avoid alcohol and caffeine, which cause fluid loss.
- **Sip warm liquids**: Chicken soup, tea, or warm apple juice can ease congestion and throat discomfort. Honey may help relieve coughing (only for children over one year and adults).

- **Get plenty of rest**: Especially important if you have a fever or severe cough. Avoid activities that leave you feeling drowsy, especially if medicated.

Other helpful measures:

- **Maintain a comfortable environment**: Use a **cool-mist humidifier** to relieve dryness and ease coughing. Clean it regularly to prevent mould or bacterial buildup.
- **Gargle with saltwater**: Mix ¼ to ½ teaspoon of salt in 4 to 8 ounces of warm water. Gargle and spit. (Not suitable for children under six.)
- **Try throat soothers**: Ice chips, lozenges, or hard candy may provide relief. Do not give these to children under six due to choking risks.
- **Use saline nasal drops or sprays**: These can moisturise nasal passages and loosen mucus.
- **For infants and young children**: Use saline drops followed by a suction bulb (inserted about ¼ to ½ inch) to gently clear mucus.
- **Consider herbal tea**: Drink **KoffHUB Herbal Tea** two to three times daily to boost immunity, soothe the throat, and support respiratory health.

References:

1. https://www.cdc.gov/antibiotic-use/colds.html
2. https://www.mayoclinic.org/diseases-conditions/common-cold/symptoms-causes/syc-20351605
3. https://share.upmc.com/2023/04/what-to-eat-when-you-have-a-cold/
4. https://www.mayoclinic.org/diseases-conditions/common-cold/diagnosis-treatment/drc-20351611

10

Constipation

Introduction

Constipation occurs when an individual has fewer than three bowel movements per week. However, bathroom habits vary widely—some people go multiple times a day, while others go only once or twice a week. Whatever your usual pattern, it is considered normal for you. A significant deviation from your routine may result in difficulty passing stool.

Common signs of constipation include:

- Dry, hard stools
- Painful bowel movements
- A lingering sensation that your bowels are not completely emptied

Causes

1. Lifestyle Factors

- Low fibre intake
- Inadequate water consumption (dehydration)
- Lack of physical activity
- Changes in routine, travel, or sleep patterns
- Excessive consumption of milk or cheese
- High levels of stress
- Ignoring the urge to have a bowel movement

2. Medications

- Strong pain relievers (narcotics)
- Nonsteroidal anti-inflammatory drugs (NSAIDs), such as ibuprofen and naproxen
- Antidepressants
- Antacids containing calcium or aluminum
- Iron supplements
- Certain allergy, blood pressure, psychiatric, and antiseizure medications

3. Medical Conditions

- Endocrine disorders (e.g., hypothyroidism, diabetes)
- Colorectal cancer
- Irritable bowel syndrome (IBS)
- Diverticulitis
- Outlet dysfunction constipation
- Obstructed defecation syndrome
- Neurologic conditions (e.g., spinal cord injuries, multiple sclerosis)
- Lazy bowel syndrome
- Intestinal pseudo-obstruction
- Structural abnormalities in the digestive tract
- Multi-organ diseases
- Pregnancy

4. Other Causes

- Slow transit of stool through the colon
- Delayed colon emptying (particularly in women or after colon surgery)
- Functional gastrointestinal disorders

- Dietary supplements and certain medications
- Changes in daily routine (e.g., aging, pregnancy, travel)
- Poor nutrition and hydration
- Low levels of physical activity

Symptoms

- **Infrequent Bowel Movements:** Fewer than three bowel movements per week
- **Hard, Dry, or Lumpy Stools:** Characterised by dry and firm consistency
- **Difficulty Passing Stools:** Pain or strain during bowel movements
- **Sensation of Incomplete Evacuation:** A feeling that stool remains in the rectum despite passing

Foods to Avoid

Avoid high-fat and low-fibre foods that can slow digestion and contribute to constipation. These include:

- Fried foods and processed meats
- Baked goods made with white flour
- Cheese and other dairy products
- Fast food and other greasy, oily meals

Fat digestion is complex and can delay gastrointestinal motility. Moreover, many high-fat foods are low in fibre, further worsening the condition.

Foods to Eat

Tips for Adequate Fibre Intake

- Adult fibre needs range from **22 to 40 grams per day**, depending on age and sex
- Older adults may struggle to consume enough fibre due to reduced appetite

- Consult a healthcare provider to create a personalised, fibre-rich meal plan
- Introduce fibre slowly to avoid gas or bloating
- Excellent sources include whole grains, legumes, vegetables, fruits, and nuts

Importance of Hydration

- Drink water, herbal teas, fruit juices, and clear broths throughout the day
- Sufficient fluid intake enhances the effectiveness of fibre
- Proper hydration softens stool, making it easier to pass
- Seek guidance from a nutritionist to determine your ideal daily fluid intake based on age, body size, activity level, and climate

Remedies

1. Stay Hydrated

- Regular water intake prevents dehydration, a major cause of constipation
- Sparkling water may be helpful, but avoid sugary or caffeinated sodas
- People with IBS may need to avoid carbonated beverages

2. Increase Fibre Intake

- Dietary fibre promotes regular bowel movements
- Soluble, non-fermentable fibre (such as psyllium) is particularly effective
- Aim for a combination of soluble and insoluble fibre
- Suggested daily intake: 35 grams for females, 40 grams for males

3. Exercise Regularly

- Physical activity stimulates digestion
- Sedentary lifestyles contribute to constipation
- Engage in walking, swimming, cycling, or jogging regularly

4. Caffeine Boost

- Coffee stimulates the muscles of the digestive tract and may help relieve constipation.
- Caffeinated coffee is generally more effective than decaffeinated.
- Consider individual tolerance, particularly in those with irritable bowel syndrome (IBS).

5. Herbal Help: Senna and Digestox Fibre

- Senna is an herbal laxative commonly used for short-term relief of constipation.
- It contains glycosides that stimulate the nerves in the gut to promote bowel movements. Senna powder is readily available in the market.
- Digestox is a soluble fibre supplement containing inulin, resistant maltodextrin, and partially hydrolysed guar gum. It is also commercially available.
- Always consult a healthcare professional before using herbal remedies, particularly if symptoms persist or if you have an underlying health condition.

References:

1. https://www.niddk.nih.gov/health-information/digestive-diseases/constipation/symptoms-causes
2. https://my.clevelandclinic.org/health/diseases/4059-constipation

3. https://www.hopkinsmedicine.org/health/wellness-and-prevention/foods-for-constipation#:~:text=move%20your%20bowels.-,Foods%20to%20Avoid%20When%20Constipated,fat%20items%20may%20be%20responsible.
4. https://www.niddk.nih.gov/health-information/digestive-diseases/constipation/eating-diet-nutrition
5. https://www.medicalnewstoday.com/articles/318694#probiotics

11

Cirrhosis

Introduction

Cirrhosis is a severe form of liver scarring that results from various liver diseases, such as hepatitis or prolonged alcohol abuse.

When the liver is injured—whether by excessive alcohol consumption or infection—it initiates a self-repair process that creates scar tissue. As cirrhosis progresses, this scarring worsens and increasingly impairs the liver's normal functions, such as detoxification and nutrient processing. In advanced stages, cirrhosis can become life-threatening.

Unfortunately, liver damage caused by cirrhosis is typically irreversible. However, early diagnosis and treatment of the underlying cause can help prevent further harm. In rare cases, timely intervention may even lead to partial reversal of the condition.

Cirrhosis, marked by liver fibrosis, often represents the final stage of chronic liver disease. With prompt medical treatment, its progression may be slowed and outcomes improved.

Causes

Cirrhosis can be caused by a variety of conditions and factors:

1. **Long-Term Alcohol Abuse**: Chronic, excessive alcohol consumption damages the liver and can lead to cirrhosis.
2. **Viral Hepatitis**: Persistent infections with hepatitis B, C, or D viruses significantly contribute to cirrhosis.

3. **Nonalcoholic Fatty Liver Disease (NAFLD):** Fat accumulation in the liver may progress to cirrhosis, especially in the inflammatory form known as nonalcoholic steatohepatitis (NASH).
4. **Hemochromatosis:** This condition involves excess iron accumulation in the body, which can lead to liver damage.
5. **Autoimmune Hepatitis:** In autoimmune hepatitis, the body's immune system attacks liver cells, potentially causing cirrhosis.
6. **Primary Biliary Cholangitis (PBC):** This disease involves progressive destruction of the bile ducts, contributing to liver scarring and cirrhosis.

Symptoms

Symptoms of cirrhosis often develop gradually. In the early stages, symptoms may be absent or nonspecific.

Early Symptoms

- Fatigue and general weakness
- Nausea and reduced appetite
- Weight loss and muscle wasting
- Redness on the palms and spider angiomas (small, dilated blood vessels visible on the upper body)

Advanced Symptoms and Complications

- Yellowing of the skin and eyes (jaundice)
- Vomiting blood
- Persistent itching
- Dark urine and tarry stools
- Easy bruising or bleeding
- Swelling in the legs (edema) or abdomen (ascites)
- Reduced libido

It is important to note that cirrhosis may remain asymptomatic until liver damage is significant. Regular check-ups and awareness of warning signs are essential for early detection and management.

Foods to Avoid

A well-managed diet plays a key role in supporting liver health. Individuals with cirrhosis should avoid:

1. **Highly Processed Foods:** Fast food, packaged snacks, canned soups, and convenience meals as they are high in hidden salt content
2. **Unhealthy Fats:** Fried foods, margarine, and vegetable shortening
3. **Salty Snacks:** Chips, pretzels, crackers, and microwave popcorn
4. **Processed Meats:** Sausages, hot dogs, bacon, deli meats, and beef jerky
5. **High-Sodium Condiments:** Soy sauce, steak sauce, teriyaki sauce, and jarred pasta sauces
6. **Undercooked or Raw Foods:** Raw or undercooked meat, poultry, eggs, fish, oysters, or mussels
7. **Alcohol:** Beer, wine, spirits, and cocktails

Avoiding these foods and beverages can reduce the strain on your liver and support better health. Consult a healthcare provider or dietitian for personalised guidance.

Foods to Eat

A liver-friendly diet focuses on whole, nutrient-rich foods that are easy for the liver to process. Recommended options include:

1. **Fruits:** Apples, oranges, pears, berries, peaches, and plums
2. **Vegetables:** Broccoli, cauliflower, asparagus, tomatoes, peas, and potatoes

3. **Protein-Rich Foods**: Eggs, dairy products, lean poultry, seafood, and plant-based proteins
4. **Legumes**: Beans, lentils, and chickpeas
5. **Nuts**: Walnuts, almonds, pistachios, cashews, and macadamias
6. **Seeds**: Chia, flax, hemp, and pumpkin seeds
7. **Whole Grains**: Brown rice, quinoa, oats, and buckwheat
8. **Heart-Healthy Fats**: Olive oil, avocado, fatty fish (e.g., salmon), nuts, and seeds
9. **Hydration**: Water, herbal tea, and coffee in moderation (if permitted by your doctor)
10. **Herbs and Spices**: Black pepper, cumin, dill, parsley, and thyme

Incorporating these foods can enhance liver function and overall well-being. Always consult a healthcare professional for individualised dietary planning.

Remedies

1. Abstain from Alcohol
    - Complete avoidance of alcohol is essential, as it significantly worsens liver damage.
2. Adopt a Low-Sodium Diet
    - Reduce salt intake to prevent fluid retention.
    - Use herbs and spices for flavour.
    - Select low-sodium versions of packaged foods.
3. Follow a Nutritious Diet
    - Prevent malnutrition with a varied and balanced diet.
    - Focus on vegetables, fruits, whole grains, and lean proteins.
    - Avoid raw or undercooked seafood.

4. Prevent Infections
    - People with cirrhosis are more vulnerable to infections.
    - Get vaccinated against hepatitis A and B, influenza, and pneumonia.
    - Practice good hygiene and avoid close contact with sick individuals.
5. Be Cautious with Medications
    - Consult your doctor before taking any medication, including over-the-counter products.
    - Avoid NSAIDs like ibuprofen and aspirin unless advised otherwise.
    - Use acetaminophen cautiously and only in recommended doses.

Following these steps can help manage cirrhosis and prevent further liver damage. Always work with your healthcare team to create a treatment plan that meets your specific needs.

References:

1. https://www.mayoclinic.org/diseases-conditions/cirrhosis/symptoms-causes/syc-20351487
2. https://www.nhs.uk/conditions/cirrhosis/
3. https://www.healthline.com/nutrition/liver-cirrhosis-diet#foods-to-eat-and-avoid
4. https://www.mayoclinic.org/diseases-conditions/cirrhosis/diagnosis-treatment/drc-20351492

12

Cancer

Introduction

Cancer is a complex disease characterised by the uncontrolled growth and spread of cells within the human body. Our bodies, composed of trillions of cells, typically follow a precise process of growth, division, and natural replacement. When cells become damaged or age, they undergo programmed cell death, making way for new, healthy cells.

In cancer, this orderly process breaks down. Abnormal or damaged cells begin to grow and divide uncontrollably, forming clusters known as tumours. Not all tumours are cancerous: some are benign and do not invade nearby tissues. In contrast, cancerous (or malignant) tumours invade surrounding tissue and can spread to distant parts of the body, a process known as metastasis.

While many cancers form solid tumours, blood-related cancers such as leukemia generally do not. Benign tumours, although noncancerous, can still pose health risks if they grow large or press on vital organs. Understanding the distinctions between benign and malignant tumours is critical for the effective diagnosis, treatment, and management of this widespread and diverse group of diseases.

Causes

Causes of Cancer: Unraveling the Genetic Roots

Cancer is, at its core, a genetic disease, arising from changes to genes that regulate how our cells grow, divide, and function.

These genetic changes—often referred to as mutations—can occur due to several factors:

1. **Errors during Cell Division**: Mistakes may occur as cells divide, leading to mutations that contribute to cancer development.
2. **Environmental Factors**: Exposure to harmful substances, such as chemicals in tobacco smoke or ultraviolet rays from the sun, can damage DNA and initiate cancer-causing mutations.
3. **Inherited Genetic Mutations**: Some people inherit mutations from their parents, which can increase their lifetime risk of certain types of cancer.

The body typically identifies and eliminates cells with damaged DNA before they become cancerous. However, this defense weakens with age, contributing to a higher risk of cancer in older adults.

Each person's cancer has a unique genetic profile, comprising a distinct combination of mutations. As a tumour grows, additional genetic changes may occur—even within the same tumour—leading to a heterogeneous cell population.

The genetic changes that drive cancer most often involve three classes of genes:

- **Proto-oncogenes** normally regulate healthy cell growth. When mutated, they can become oncogenes, promoting uncontrolled cell proliferation.
- **Tumour suppressor genes** help regulate cell division. Mutations in these genes can allow cells to divide uncontrollably.
- **DNA repair genes** fix damaged DNA. Mutations in these genes hinder DNA repair, allowing additional mutations to accumulate and drive cancer progression.

As research advances, scientists have identified common mutations across many types of cancer. These discoveries have led to the development of targeted therapies that act on specific genetic changes, offering more precise treatments that may be effective regardless of the cancer's origin.

Symptoms

While many signs and symptoms do not indicate cancer, persistent or worsening changes should not be ignored. Early medical evaluation can help determine whether symptoms are cancer-related or due to another condition, enabling timely and appropriate intervention.

Below are common signs and symptoms that may be associated with cancer. However, they can also result from noncancerous conditions:

1. **Fatigue**: Persistent, unexplained tiredness that does not improve with rest
2. **Unexplained Weight Changes**: Significant weight loss or gain (typically 10 pounds or more) without a known cause
3. **Eating Problems**: Loss of appetite, difficulty swallowing, persistent nausea or vomiting, or abdominal pain
4. **Swelling or Lumps**: Noticeable lumps or swellings anywhere in the body
5. **Breast or Body Abnormalities**: Thickening or lumps in the breast or other areas of the body
6. **Persistent Pain**: New or unusual pain that does not resolve
7. **Skin Changes**: Unexplained bleeding or scaling lumps, new moles or changes in existing moles, nonhealing sores, or yellowing of the skin or eyes (jaundice)
8. **Respiratory Issues**: Chronic cough or hoarseness that persists

9. **Bleeding or Bruising**: Unexplained bleeding or bruising without injury
10. **Changes in Bowel or Bladder Habits**: Persistent constipation or diarrhea, changes in stool appearance, blood in the urine, frequent urination, or pain during urination
11. **Fever or Night Sweats**: Unexplained fevers or drenching night sweats
12. **Headaches**: Persistent or severe headaches without an obvious cause
13. **Vision or Hearing Changes**: Altered or reduced vision or hearing that does not resolve
14. **Mouth Changes**: Sores, bleeding, pain, or numbness in the mouth that persists

While these symptoms can be linked to cancer, many are also associated with less serious conditions. Nonetheless, it is essential to consult a physician if you notice any unusual or persistent changes in your health. Early detection significantly increases the likelihood of successful treatment.

Foods to Avoid

Maintaining awareness of what you consume is crucial during cancer treatment. Whenever possible, prepare meals at home, read nutrition labels, and avoid certain types of food. Highly refined and processed foods, along with fried items containing inflammatory hydrogenated oils, should be eliminated from the diet.

Given the immune system's potential vulnerability during cancer treatment, it is advisable to avoid foods that pose a risk of foodborne illness. These include:

1. **Lightly Cooked or Raw Fish**: Avoid sushi and raw or undercooked fish.

2. **Soft-Cooked Eggs and Foods Containing Raw Eggs:** Avoid items such as homemade mayonnaise or salad dressings made with raw eggs.
3. **Unpasteurised Cheeses and Dairy Products:** Choose only pasteurised cheeses and dairy to prevent exposure to harmful bacteria.
4. **Unwashed Fruits and Vegetables:** Wash all produce thoroughly to reduce the risk of contamination.

By making informed dietary choices, you support your immune system and contribute positively to the effectiveness of your cancer treatment.

Foods to Eat

Adopting a health-conscious diet can significantly support your well-being during cancer treatment. Consider the following dietary adjustments—particularly if you have a chronic illness—to strengthen your body before and during treatment:

1. **Plant-Based Proteins**
    - Include a variety of vegetables, beans, legumes, nuts, and seeds in your meals.
    - If consuming animal products, opt for lean proteins such as chicken or fish.
    - These foods are rich in essential vitamins and minerals crucial for health and recovery.
2. **Healthy Fats**
    - Incorporate monounsaturated and polyunsaturated fats for their anti-inflammatory benefits.
    - Good sources include avocados, olive oil, grapeseed oil, and walnuts, all high in omega-3 fatty acids.
    - Omega-3s help reduce inflammation and support heart health.

3. **Healthy Carbohydrates**
    - Choose minimally processed whole grains such as whole wheat, bran, and oats.
    - These contain soluble fibre that promotes a healthy gut microbiome and supports cellular repair and metabolic function.
4. **Vitamins and Minerals**
    - Include foods fortified with vitamin D—such as milk, yogurt, orange juice, and fortified cereals.
    - Micronutrients play essential roles in enzyme activity, immune response, and inflammation reduction.

Making proactive, nourishing dietary choices empowers your body with the nutrients it needs to remain resilient during cancer treatment.

Remedies

Herbs for Natural Cancer Support

1. **Turmeric**
    - *Active Ingredient*: Curcumin
    - *Properties*: Anti-inflammatory and antioxidant
    - *Benefits*: May reduce inflammation and inhibit tumour growth
2. **Ginger**
    - *Benefits*: Known to alleviate nausea, vomiting, and pain during treatment
3. **Cayenne Pepper**
    - *Active Compound*: Capsaicin
    - *Effect*: May induce apoptosis (programmed cell death) in cancer cells

4. **Garlic**
    - *Benefits*: May reduce tumour growth and protect healthy cells from chemotherapy damage
5. **Echinacea**
    - *Traditional Use*: Immune booster and infection fighter
    - *Recent Studies*: Supports immune system function
6. **Ginkgo**
    - *Active Compounds*: Ginkgolides
    - *Properties*: Anti-inflammatory, antioxidant, and potentially anticancer
7. **Ginseng**
    - *Benefits*: May reduce inflammation, inhibit tumour growth, and protect healthy cells

Supplements for Cancer Support

1. **Omega-3 Fatty Acids**: Role: Reduces inflammation and supports cardiovascular health.
2. **Vitamin D**: Benefits: Supports immune function; low levels are linked to increased cancer risk. Low vitamin D levels have been associated with increased risk of certain cancers and may be linked to reduced risk of advanced cancer development.
3. **Probiotics**: Effects: Improve digestive health and immune system performance.
4. **Antioxidants**: Benefits: Reduce inflammation and protect cells from oxidative damage.
5. **Selenium**: Benefits: Neutralises free radicals and prevents cellular damage.
6. **Zinc**: Role: Supports immune function and may have anticancer properties.

7. **Vitamin E**: Role: Acts as an antioxidant to protect cells from damage.

Final Note

Exploring the use of herbs and supplements can offer a complementary approach to conventional cancer treatment. However, these remedies should be integrated with care. Always consult your oncologist or healthcare provider before introducing new herbs or dietary supplements, especially during treatment. This ensures safety and avoids interactions with prescribed therapies.

References:

1. https://www.cancer.gov/about-cancer/understanding/what-is-cancer
2. https://www.cancer.org/cancer/diagnosis-staging/signs-and-symptoms-of-cancer.html
3. https://www.hopkinsmedicine.org/health/conditions-and-diseases/cancer/cancer-diet-foods-to-add-and-avoid-during-cancer-treatment
4. https://www.patientpower.info/navigating-cancer/natural-remedies-cancer

13

Cough

Introduction

Coughing is the body's natural reflex to clear irritants from the upper (throat) and lower (lungs) airways. It serves as a vital mechanism to aid healing and protect the respiratory system.

Types of Cough

Categorised by Duration:

1. **Acute Cough**: Begins suddenly and typically lasts two to three weeks.
2. **Subacute Cough**: Persists beyond an infection, lasting three to eight weeks.
3. **Chronic Cough**: Lasts more than eight weeks; also referred to as a persistent cough.
4. **Refractory Cough**: A chronic cough that is resistant to treatment.

Categorised by Mucus Production:

1. **Productive Cough (Wet Cough)**: Produces mucus or phlegm.
2. **Non-Productive Cough (Dry Cough)**: Does not produce mucus or phlegm.

Categorised by Sound and Condition:

1. **Whooping Cough**: Associated with a pertussis infection, characterised by a distinctive "whooping" sound.

2. **Barking Cough**: Resembles a barking sound; often indicative of croup.
3. **Wheezing Cough**: Associated with blocked airways and conditions such as asthma or the common cold.

Categorised by Timing:

1. **Daytime Cough**: Occurs primarily during the day.
2. **Nighttime (Nocturnal) Cough**: Occurs primarily at night.
3. **Cough with Vomiting**: Common in children; intense coughing can lead to gagging and occasional vomiting.

Causes

Coughing is a common physiological response triggered by a variety of factors. From everyday irritants to underlying health conditions, understanding the underlying cause is essential for effective treatment.

Irritants or Allergens:

- Smoke
- Strong smells (e.g., cleaners, perfumes)
- Mold
- Dust
- Pollen
- Pet dander

Medications:

- Certain medications, such as ACE inhibitors (used to treat high blood pressure), may trigger coughing.

Common Causes of Acute and Subacute Cough:

- Cold
- Flu
- Acute bronchitis or bronchiolitis

- Sinusitis
- Pneumonia
- Whooping cough (pertussis)
- Asthma
- Allergies
- Exposure to secondhand or thirdhand smoke

Common Causes of Chronic Cough:

- Chronic bronchitis
- Asthma
- Allergies
- Chronic obstructive pulmonary disease (COPD)
- Gastroesophageal reflux disease (GERD) is a chronic digestive disorder in which stomach contents and acid frequently flow back into the oesophagus.
- Throat disorders, including vocal cord issues
- Postnasal drip
- Heart failure and other cardiac conditions

Symptoms

When associated with a chronic cough, various signs and symptoms may be present, including:

Nasal Symptoms:

- Persistent runny or congested nose

Throat-Related Sensations:

- Postnasal drip (sensation of liquid trickling down the throat)
- Frequent throat clearing
- Sore throat

Voice Changes:

- Hoarseness or other changes in vocal quality

Respiratory Issues:

- Wheezing
- Shortness of breath

Digestive Symptoms:

- Heartburn
- Sour taste in the mouth

Less Common:

- Rarely coughing up blood

These symptoms can provide insight into the complexity of the condition and help guide accurate diagnosis and treatment.

Foods to Avoid

1. **Dairy Products:** Avoid milk, ice cream, and cheese during a cold, as these may worsen nasal congestion.
2. **Caffeine and Alcohol:** These can dehydrate the body and impair immune function, potentially prolonging symptoms.
3. **Fried Foods:** Deep-fried items may exacerbate cough conditions and should be replaced with healthier alternatives.
4. **Histamine-Rich Foods:** Avoid foods such as avocados, mushrooms, and alcohol, which can trigger excess mucus production.
5. **Sugary Foods:** Limit sugar intake, as it may promote inflammation and worsen symptoms of cough and cold.

Foods to Eat

1. **Chicken Soup:** Offers anti-inflammatory properties and essential nutrients that aid recovery.

2. **Citrus Fruits**: Oranges, lemons, and other citrus fruits are rich in vitamin C and can help reduce cold symptoms.
3. **Green Vegetables and Antioxidant-Rich Foods**: Foods like broccoli, kale, green tea, red onions, and blueberries offer antibacterial effects and supply vital nutrients.
4. **Spicy Foods**: Foods containing capsaicin (e.g., chilli peppers) may relieve nasal congestion but should be consumed in moderation if experiencing digestive discomfort.
5. **Ginger**: Ginger tea soothes sore throats and decongests the respiratory system. It also possesses anti-nausea, antioxidant, antimicrobial, and anticancer properties.
6. **Garlic**: Known for its immune-boosting effects; add to soups or broths for antibacterial, antiviral, and antifungal benefits.
7. **Coconut Water**: Helps prevent dehydration and replenishes glucose and electrolytes.
8. **Honey**: Has antimicrobial properties. Mix with warm milk, water, or tea for a soothing effect on the throat.
9. **Bananas**: Easy to digest, nutrient-rich, and contain soluble fibre that supports digestion during illness.
10. **Dark Green Vegetables**: Packed with essential vitamins and anti-inflammatory compounds that help protect cells and support recovery.

Remedies

1. **Honey**: Research supports honey's effectiveness in relieving cough—sometimes more so than over-the-counter options. A spoonful in hot herbal tea can provide relief.
2. **Ginger**: A 2015 study and traditional use both support its role in easing dry or asthmatic coughs. Often consumed in dishes or tea. Individuals prone to stomach issues should use with caution.

3. **Hot Fluids**: A 2008 study showed that warm liquids relieve cough, runny nose, and sneezing. Clear broths, herbal teas, and decaffeinated black tea may ease sore throats and chills.
4. **Steam Inhalation**: Useful for wet coughs with mucus. Inhaling steam—via a hot shower or a bowl of hot water with herbs or eucalyptus oil—can provide respiratory relief within 10–15 minutes.
5. **Marshmallow Root**: Contains mucilage, which coats the throat and alleviates irritation. A 2020 in vitro study highlighted its anti-inflammatory and antioxidant effects. Can be consumed as a tea.
6. **Saltwater Gargle**: A time-tested remedy that helps loosen mucus and ease sore throat symptoms. Mix ½ teaspoon of salt in warm water and gargle several times daily. Not recommended for children or individuals with high blood pressure.

References:

1. https://my.clevelandclinic.org/health/symptoms/17755-cough
2. https://www.mayoclinic.org/diseases-conditions/chronic-cough/symptoms-causes/syc-20351575
3. https://www.pristyncare.com/blog/foods-to-eat-and-avoid-cough/
4. https://www.medicalnewstoday.com/articles/322394#natural-cough-remedies

14

Cramps

Introduction

A muscle cramp is a sudden, often painful tightening of a muscle, commonly referred to as a "charley horse." These cramps can occur during physical activity, strenuous work, or even in warm conditions. Certain medications or medical conditions may also trigger them.

The good news is that muscle cramps are generally not serious. Most can be managed at home with simple self-care strategies.

Causes

1. Muscle cramps may result from overexertion, prolonged static positioning, or excessive sweating. In some cases, the cause remains unknown.
2. Some cramps are associated with medical conditions, such as:
    - Reduced blood flow due to narrowed leg arteries, often occurring during exercise
    - Nerve compression in the spine, with pain worsening while walking
3. A deficiency in dietary minerals—such as potassium, calcium, or magnesium—can contribute to leg cramps. Diuretics used for managing high blood pressure may exacerbate this by increasing mineral loss through urination.

Symptoms

1. **Location:** Most often occur in the legs, particularly the calves.
2. **Duration:** Cramps typically last a few seconds to several minutes.
3. **Aftereffects:** Soreness may persist for hours or even days after the episode.

Foods to Avoid

1. **Processed Foods:** Limit consumption of fast food and packaged snacks, which may lack essential nutrients.
2. **Low-Nutrient Options:** Avoid foods that contribute to electrolyte imbalance due to poor nutritional value.

Foods to Eat

1. **Milk:** Rich in calcium and vitamin D, both essential for muscle health
2. **Leafy Greens:** High in potassium; includes spinach, kale, Swiss chard, and collard greens
3. **Bone Broth:** Hydrating and abundant in electrolytes (potassium, calcium, magnesium, and sodium)
4. **Seeds and Nuts:** Excellent sources of magnesium; try pumpkin seeds, chia seeds, almonds, cashews, and peanuts
5. **Bananas:** Contain potassium, sodium, magnesium, and calcium, along with fibre and key vitamins
6. **Avocados:** Provide potassium, healthy fats, calcium, magnesium, and sodium
7. **Olives:** Replenish sodium lost through sweating and offer other key electrolytes
8. **Tomatoes:** Contain potassium, calcium, sodium, and magnesium; also high in lycopene, an antioxidant

9. **Salmon:** A cold-water fish rich in beneficial minerals and omega-3 fatty acids
10. **Melons:** Hydrating and mineral-rich (calcium, potassium, magnesium, sodium)
11. **Sweet Potatoes:** Composed of about 80% water; high in potassium, vitamin C, and fibre
12. **Coconut Water:** A natural electrolyte beverage, particularly high in sodium
13. **Electrolyte Drinks:** Ideal for replenishing minerals during or after heavy sweating; choose options without added sugar
14. **Beans:** High in phosphorus, important for muscle function; varieties include black, navy, pinto, kidney, red, and Great Northern
15. **Yogurt:** Offers calcium, phosphorus, magnesium, sodium, and potassium; opt for unsweetened varieties

Remedies

1. **Stretch and Massage:**
    - Gently stretch the affected muscle and massage the area to reduce tension.
2. **Calf Cramp Relief:**
    - Keep the leg straight and pull the toes toward your face.
    - Stand on the cramped leg and apply gentle pressure.
    - For a back thigh cramp, standing stretches can help.
3. **Front Thigh Cramp Relief:**
    - Pull the foot of the cramped side toward your buttock while holding a chair for balance.
4. **Heat or Cold Application:**
    - Use a warm towel, heating pad, or take a hot shower to relax tight muscles.

5. **Warm baths can also provide relief.**
    - Alternatively, apply an ice pack to the sore area to ease discomfort.

References:

1. https://www.mayoclinic.org/diseases-conditions/muscle-cramp/symptoms-causes/syc-20350820
2. https://www.healthline.com/health/pain-relief/what-causes-leg-cramps#symptoms
3. https://www.health.com/foods-that-prevent-muscle-cramps-7973949#:~:text=Foods%20to%20Avoid,be%20low%20in%20nutritional%20value.
4. https://www.mayoclinic.org/diseases-conditions/muscle-cramp/diagnosis-treatment/drc-20350825#:~:text=Apply%20heat%20or%20cold.,ice%20also%20might%20relieve%20pain.

15

Cervical

Introduction

Neck pain, or **cervicalgia**, refers to discomfort in or around the cervical spine—the portion of the spine located just beneath the head. It is a common symptom linked to a variety of injuries and medical conditions. Common causes include cervical spondylosis, muscle strain and nerve compression.

Neck pain may be **axial** (confined to the neck) or **radicular** (radiating into areas such as the shoulders or arms). It may be classified as **acute** (lasting from a few days to six weeks) or **chronic** (persisting for more than three months).

When untreated, neck pain can significantly interfere with daily activities and reduce quality of life. Fortunately, most cases are not serious and can be effectively managed through conservative approaches such as pain management, exercise, and stress relief.

Causes

1. **Aging**: Natural wear and tear over time can cause degeneration of cervical spine structures, resulting in conditions like osteoarthritis or spinal stenosis.
2. **Physical Strain**: Overuse of neck muscles during repetitive or strenuous activities—particularly when combined with poor posture from prolonged desk work, handheld device use, or weak abdominal support—can place excessive stress on the cervical spine and surrounding muscles, leading to stiffness and pain.

3. **Mental Stress:** Chronic stress may cause individuals to unknowingly tighten their neck muscles, resulting in pain and stiffness.
4. **Injury:** Accidents or trauma may injure muscles, ligaments, intervertebral discs, joints, or nerve roots. Whiplash from car accidents is a typical example.
5. **Growths:** Tumours, cysts, or bone spurs may exert pressure on nerves in the neck, resulting in pain.
6. **Other Health Conditions:** Neck pain may also be a symptom of underlying medical issues such as meningitis, rheumatoid arthritis, or cancer.

Symptoms

1. **Neck Pain:** Discomfort that may radiate to the shoulders or arms
2. **Headaches:** Often associated with cervical spondylosis
3. **Grinding Sensation:** A creaking or grinding noise during neck movement
4. **Weakness:** Particularly in the arms or legs
5. **Numbness:** In the shoulders, arms, or hands
6. **Stiff Neck:** Reduced range of motion or difficulty turning the head
7. **Balance Issues:** Difficulty maintaining stability while walking
8. **Bladder or Bowel Problems:** In rare cases, loss of control over bladder or bowel function

Foods to Avoid

1. **Sour Foods (Especially Curd):** Strictly avoid sour items, with curd being a primary item to exclude.
2. **Fried Foods and Pulses:** Refrain from consuming fried items and pulse-based preparations.

3. **Highly Acidic Foods:** Red meat, citrus fruits, and white potatoes can increase acidity in the body, potentially exacerbating joint inflammation.
4. **Excessive Protein:** Diets overly high in protein may hinder calcium absorption. Avoid excessive intake of salt, phosphorus (often found in carbonated drinks), caffeine, and alcohol, as these can interfere with calcium levels.

Foods to Eat

1. **Bitter Vegetables:** Include bitter drumstick, neem flowers, and bitter gourd in your diet.
2. **Vitamin A- and C-Rich Foods:** Fresh fruits and vegetables rich in these vitamins offer natural anti-inflammatory effects.
3. **Omega-3 Fatty Acids and Vitamin E:** Found in oilseeds, nuts, and fatty fish, these nutrients help reduce inflammation.
4. **Frequent, Smaller Meals:** Eat four to six smaller meals daily instead of three large ones to improve digestion and nutrient absorption.
5. **Moderate Protein and Salt Intake:** Avoid diets overly rich in protein. Minimise salt, carbonated drinks (high in phosphorus), caffeine, and alcohol to support calcium retention.

Remedies

1. **Heat Therapy:** Take a hot shower or apply a heating pad (on the lowest setting) to the affected area for 15 minutes every few hours. Heat helps relax muscles and promote blood circulation.
2. **Cold Therapy:** Apply an ice pack or a bag of frozen vegetables wrapped in a thin towel for 15 minutes. This reduces swelling and inflammation. Cold therapy is especially useful immediately following an injury.

3. **Exercise:** Follow your healthcare provider's recommended neck exercises to relieve pain and improve flexibility. Avoid exercise in cases of severe neck injury or a pinched nerve.
4. **Stress Reduction:** Incorporate practices such as mindfulness, meditation, deep breathing exercises, and yoga to reduce overall muscular tension.
5. **Quit Smoking:** Smoking deteriorates bone structure, worsens degenerative disc disease, and delays healing. Quitting can substantially benefit cervical spine health.
6. **Hydration:** Staying well hydrated supports muscle function and helps reduce stiffness.

Persistent or worsening cervical pain should be evaluated by a healthcare professional to rule out serious underlying conditions.

References:

1. https://my.clevelandclinic.org/health/symptoms/21179-neck-pain
2. https://www.hopkinsmedicine.org/health/conditions-and-diseases/cervical-spondylosis
3. https://www.bhagwatiayurveda.com/cervical-spondylosis/#:~:text=Sour%20things%2C%20particularly%20curd%2C%20are,in%20a%20cervical%20spondylosis%20diet.

16

Diabetes

Introduction

Diabetes is a condition marked by elevated blood glucose (sugar) levels and represents a significant public health concern. It impairs the body's ability to use glucose for energy. Glucose—derived from food and produced internally by the body—is regulated by insulin, a hormone made by the pancreas.

In individuals with diabetes, either the body does not produce sufficient insulin or fails to use it effectively. This leads to high blood glucose levels, which can cause various complications, including damage to the eyes, kidneys, nerves, and heart. Additionally, diabetes is associated with an increased risk of certain cancers.

The three primary types of diabetes are **Type 1, Type 2,** and **gestational diabetes:**

- **Type 1 diabetes** involves insufficient insulin production and is often diagnosed in children or young adults.
- **Type 2 diabetes,** the most common form, is characterised by the body's inability to use insulin properly. It is frequently associated with overweight, obesity, and family history.
- **Gestational diabetes** develops during pregnancy and usually resolves after childbirth but raises the risk of developing Type 2 diabetes later in life.

Prediabetes—a condition in which blood glucose levels are higher than normal but not yet in the diabetic range—also increases the risk of Type 2 diabetes and heart disease.

Less common forms include **monogenic diabetes**, caused by a single gene mutation, and diabetes due to **pancreatic damage** from conditions such as cystic fibrosis, pancreatitis, or pancreatic surgery.

Understanding the different types and causes of diabetes is critical to preventing or managing the condition and reducing the risk of complications.

Causes

Type 1 Diabetes

- **Immune System Response**: The body's immune system mistakenly destroys insulin-producing beta cells in the pancreas.
- **Genetic and Environmental Triggers**: A combination of genetic predisposition and possible environmental factors (such as viral infections) may initiate the disease.

Type 2 Diabetes

- **Lifestyle and Genetic Factors**: Overweight, obesity, physical inactivity, and family history significantly increase risk.
- **Insulin Resistance**: Insulin is a hormone produced by the pancreas that helps cells absorb glucose from the blood for energy. In diabetes, this process is disrupted, leading to high blood sugar levels because the body's cells do not respond properly to insulin. At first, the pancreas compensates by producing more insulin, but over time it cannot sustain this increased output.

Gestational Diabetes

- **Hormonal Changes in Pregnancy**: Pregnancy hormones can cause insulin resistance.
- **Risk Factors**: Being overweight, obese, or having a family history of diabetes increases the likelihood of developing gestational diabetes.

Other Causes

Genetic Mutations: A single gene mutation can cause monogenic diabetes.

Diseases: Conditions such as cystic fibrosis, hemochromatosis, and hormonal disorders may lead to diabetes.

Pancreatic Damage: Pancreatitis, pancreatic cancer, physical trauma, or surgical removal of the pancreas can impair insulin production.

Medications: Certain drugs—such as niacin, diuretics, anti-seizure medications, and statins—may interfere with insulin secretion or action.

Symptoms

- **Increased Thirst and Urination**: Frequent urination and excessive thirst are common signs of high blood glucose.
- **Increased Hunger**: Persistent, unexplained feelings of hunger.
- **Fatigue**: Ongoing tiredness or lack of energy.
- **Blurred Vision**: Difficulty seeing clearly due to fluid shifts in the eyes.
- **Numbness or Tingling**: A tingling or numb sensation in the hands or feet.
- **Slow-Healing Sores**: Cuts, wounds, or ulcers that heal slowly.

- **Unexplained Weight Loss:** Significant weight loss without a change in diet or activity.
- **Onset Patterns:**
    - **Type 1 diabetes** typically develops rapidly over a few weeks.
    - **Type 2 diabetes** develops gradually over several years, often with mild or unnoticed symptoms.
- **Asymptomatic Cases:** Type 2 diabetes may go undetected until complications such as vision problems or cardiovascular issues arise.

Foods to Avoid

Limit or Avoid:

1. **Fried and High-Saturated Fat Foods:** Foods rich in saturated and trans fats (e.g., deep-fried items, processed snacks, fast food).
2. **High-Sodium Foods:** Items with excessive salt, such as processed meats, pickles, and canned soups.
3. **Sweets and Sugary Treats:** Baked goods, candies, pastries, ice cream, and similar high-sugar desserts.
4. **Sugar-Sweetened Beverages:** Regular sodas, energy drinks, and fruit juices with added sugar.

Hydration Choices:

Water over Sugary Drinks:

- Choose water instead of sweetened beverages.
- Consider sugar substitutes in coffee or tea.

Alcohol in Moderation:

Recommended Limits:

- Women: Up to one drink per day.
- Men: Up to two drinks per day.

Precautions for People on Medication:

- Alcohol may cause hypoglycemia (low blood sugar) in individuals using insulin or insulin-stimulating medications.
- It is advisable to consume alcohol with food, especially if there has been a delay between meals.

Foods to Eat

1. Variety Is Key:

- Incorporate a wide range of nutritious foods from all food groups.

2. Vegetables:

- Non-starchy: Broccoli, carrots, leafy greens, bell peppers, tomatoes.
- Starchy: Potatoes, corn, green peas (consume in moderation).

3. Fruits:

- Oranges, melons, berries, apples, bananas, grapes (prefer whole fruits over juices).

4. Grains:

- Make at least half your grain intake whole grains.
- Examples include wheat, brown rice, oats, cornmeal, barley, and quinoa.

5. Protein:

- Lean meats, skinless chicken or turkey, fish, eggs.
- Plant-based proteins: nuts, peanuts, lentils, chickpeas, split peas, tofu, and soy-based meat alternatives.

6. Dairy:

- Choose non-fat or low-fat options.
- Includes milk, lactose-free milk, yoghurt, and cheese.

7. Heart-Healthy Fats:

- Use oils such as canola, olive, or sunflower.
- Include nuts, seeds, avocados, and fatty fish like salmon, tuna, and mackerel.

8. Cooking Choices:

- Use plant-based oils instead of butter, cream, lard, shortening, or stick margarine.

Note: Your diabetes meal plan, developed in consultation with your healthcare team, can include your favourite foods—enjoyed in moderation and with balance.

Remedies

1. Stress Management:

- Managing stress is essential for blood sugar control.
- Try deep breathing, walking, meditation, regular exercise, or engaging in hobbies.
- Speak with a mental health professional if needed.
- Discuss stress management strategies with your doctor for personalised support.

2. Healthy Eating:

- Consult a doctor or nutritionist to create an effective meal plan.
- Include high-fibre foods such as whole grains, fruits, and vegetables.
- Prioritise water over sugary beverages.
- Follow recommended dietary changes carefully for optimal results.

3. Exercise:

- Engage in regular physical activity under medical guidance.

- Exercise helps regulate blood sugar, promotes weight loss, and improves overall health.
- Begin with light activities like walking and gradually incorporate yoga or strength training.
- Always consult a healthcare professional before starting a new exercise routine.

4. Onion:

- Studies suggest that onions may help lower blood sugar levels.
- Dried onion powder and bioactive compounds in onions have shown potential benefits.
- Onion juice has demonstrated glucose-lowering effects in some clinical studies.
- Consult an Ayurvedic or allopathic physician before use.

5. Bel (Bengal Quince):

- Leaves of the bel tree may help lower blood sugar, urea, and cholesterol.
- May help prevent sudden spikes in blood glucose after meals.
- Use under medical supervision.

6. Neem:

- Animal studies indicate neem may reduce blood sugar levels.
- It may enhance glucose uptake by cells and promote glycogen storage.
- Human studies are limited; consult a doctor before use.

7. Babul (Acacia arabica):

- Babul seeds, widely found in India, may have anti-diabetic effects.

- Animal research shows potential for supporting insulin release.
- Further research is required. Always consult your doctor before use.

8. Aloe Vera:

- Animal studies suggest aloe vera may lower blood glucose and improve insulin secretion.
- May enhance cellular glucose usage.
- Human evidence is still emerging—seek medical advice before using aloe vera for diabetes.

References:

1. https://www.niddk.nih.gov/health-information/diabetes/overview/preventing-problems
2. https://pharmeasy.in/blog/home-remedies-for-diabetes/

17

Diarrhoea

Introduction

Diarrhoea—a common yet disruptive gastrointestinal condition—is defined as the passage of three or more loose or liquid stools in a single day, exceeding normal frequency, volume, or water content. A frequent cause is viral gastroenteritis, or "stomach flu," which often resolves on its own within a few days. However, the range of causes extends far beyond this typical scenario.

While many cases of diarrhoea are mild and self-limiting, some can become severe and require hospitalisation. This article focuses on diarrhoea in adults and individuals aged twelve and above. For information on diarrhoea in infants and young children, refer to a separate resource.

Characterised by loose, watery, and sometimes more frequent bowel movements, diarrhoea can occur alone or be accompanied by symptoms such as nausea, vomiting, abdominal pain, and weight loss. Although most episodes are acute and brief, persistent diarrhoea lasting several weeks may indicate a more serious underlying condition. These may include irritable bowel syndrome (IBS), prolonged infections, celiac disease, or inflammatory bowel disease (IBD).

A clear understanding of diarrhoea—its forms, causes, and implications—is essential for effective diagnosis, management, and treatment.

Causes

Diarrhoea can result from a wide range of triggers, including infections, food intolerances, medications, and underlying digestive disorders. Below is an overview of common causes:

1. Viral Infections: Numerous viruses can cause diarrhoea, including Norwalk virus (norovirus), enteric adenoviruses, astrovirus, cytomegalovirus, and the virus responsible for COVID-19. In children, rotavirus is a leading cause of acute diarrhoea.

2. Bacterial and Parasitic Infections: Bacteria such as Escherichia coli (E. coli), Salmonella, and Shigella, as well as parasites like Giardia, may be ingested through contaminated food or water—particularly during international travel (commonly referred to as traveller's diarrhoea). Clostridioides difficile (C. diff) is another notable bacterium that can cause diarrhoea, especially following antibiotic use or hospitalisation.

3. Medications: Several medications can induce diarrhoea. Antibiotics, in particular, may disrupt the natural balance of gut flora. Other culprits include anti-cancer drugs, magnesium-containing antacids, and certain heart or blood pressure medications.

4. Lactose Intolerance: Individuals with lactose intolerance lack sufficient lactase—the enzyme needed to digest lactose, the sugar found in dairy products. This often leads to diarrhoea following the consumption of milk, cheese, or ice cream. The condition tends to worsen with age.

5. Fructose Sensitivity: Fructose, a sugar found naturally in fruits and honey and commonly added to sweetened beverages, can trigger diarrhoea in individuals who have difficulty digesting it.

6. Artificial Sweeteners: Sugar substitutes such as sorbitol, erythritol, and mannitol—often found in sugar-free gum, candies, and diet foods—can cause diarrhoea, even in healthy individuals.

7. Surgical Interventions: Surgeries involving partial removal of the intestines or gallbladder may alter digestive processes and lead to diarrhoea.

8. Chronic Digestive Disorders: Persistent diarrhoea can be a symptom of chronic gastrointestinal conditions, including:

- Irritable bowel syndrome (IBS)
- Crohn's disease
- Ulcerative colitis
- Celiac disease
- Microscopic colitis
- Small intestinal bacterial overgrowth (SIBO)

Understanding diarrhoea involves recognising its underlying mechanism: an imbalance in water absorption and secretion within the intestines. This imbalance results in stools that contain too much liquid, either due to insufficient absorption or excessive fluid secretion. Identifying the specific cause is key to managing and treating the condition effectively.

Short-Term Causes

- **Infections:** Viral gastroenteritis, waterborne parasites, and bacteria that cause food poisoning.
- **Dietary Factors:** Sudden dietary changes, consumption of certain ingredients, artificial sweeteners, and excessive alcohol intake.
- **Stress:** Psychological stress can contribute to short-term episodes of diarrhoea.

Long-Term Causes

- **Chronic Conditions:** Inflammatory bowel disease (Crohn's disease and ulcerative colitis), irritable bowel syndrome (IBS), food intolerances, diverticulitis, malabsorption syndromes, and chronic constipation.

- **Immunocompromised Individuals**: People with weakened immune systems—such as those undergoing cancer treatment, living with HIV/AIDS, or recovering from organ transplantation—may experience prolonged diarrhoea following gastroenteritis.

Symptoms

Diarrhoea, typically marked by frequent loose or watery stools, is often accompanied by a range of other symptoms, including:

1. **Abdominal Cramps or Pain**: Cramping or discomfort in the belly is a common feature.

2. **Bloating**: A feeling of abdominal fullness or swelling.

3. **Nausea**: Often precedes or accompanies diarrhoea.

4. **Vomiting**: May occur alongside other symptoms.

5. **Fever**: Indicates an underlying infection in some cases.

6. **Blood in the Stool**: A potential sign of more serious gastrointestinal issues.

7. **Mucus in the Stool**: May be present with certain infections or inflammatory conditions.

8. **Urgency**: A sudden, compelling need for a bowel movement, often difficult to control.

Foods to Avoid

To support recovery and minimise gastrointestinal irritation, avoid the following:

1. **Fried and Greasy Foods**: These can worsen symptoms and prolong recovery.

2. **Gas-Producing Fruits and Vegetables**: Limit broccoli, peppers, beans, peas, berries, prunes, chickpeas, leafy greens, and corn.

3. **Caffeine, Alcohol, and Carbonated Beverages**: These can irritate the digestive system and contribute to dehydration.

4. Dairy Products: If lactose intolerant or sensitive, reduce intake of milk, cheese, and cream, especially during active symptoms.

Foods to Eat

Choose easy-to-digest, low-fibre, and nutrient-supportive options during recovery:

1. Lean Protein:

- Baked or broiled meats: beef, pork, chicken, turkey, or fish.
- Cooked eggs and low-fat dairy (if tolerated), such as milk, cheese, or yogurt.

2. Refined Grains:

- White bread, white rice, pasta, cream of wheat, cornflakes, and oatmeal.
- Pancakes and waffles made with refined white flour (avoid high-sugar toppings like syrup or honey).

3. Cooked Vegetables:

- Carrots, green beans, mushrooms, beets, peeled zucchini, asparagus tips, and acorn squash.
- Bake or steam vegetables; remove seeds and skins when possible.
- Baked potatoes without skins are also gentle on the digestive tract.

4. Light Desserts and Snacks (in moderation):

- Fruit-flavoured gelatin, ice pops, plain cakes, cookies, and sherbet.

Remedies

1. Hydration:

- Replenish lost fluids with water, broth, or oral rehydration solutions (ORS).
- For children, use pediatric electrolyte solutions.
- Avoid alcohol, caffeinated beverages, and dairy products during active symptoms.

2. Probiotics:

- Support gut flora with probiotic-rich foods like yogurt, kefir, kimchi, and sauerkraut.
- Consider probiotic supplements (e.g., Saccharomyces boulardii) under medical supervision.

3. BRAT Diet:

- The BRAT diet—Bananas, Rice, Applesauce, Toast—is a well-known short-term dietary approach to help stabilise stools.
- Additional low-fibre, bland foods include boiled potatoes, cooked cereals, and skinless chicken.

4. Foods to Avoid (Reiterated):

- High-fibre foods (bran, raw fruits, and vegetables).
- Common irritants: alcohol, artificial sweeteners, beans, berries, broccoli, cabbage, coffee, and dairy (if sensitive).

Note: Seek immediate medical attention if symptoms are severe, persistent (lasting more than two days in adults), or include concerning signs such as blood in the stool, high fever, dehydration, or significant weight loss. In children, prompt consultation with a healthcare provider is especially important.

References:

1. https://www.mayoclinic.org/diseases-conditions/diarrhea/symptoms-causes/syc-20352241
2. https://www.healthdirect.gov.au/diarrhoea#:~:text=Diarrhoea%20is%20when%20more%20than,lasting%20for%20over%20four%20weeks.
3. https://medlineplus.gov/ency/patientinstructions/000121.htm#:~:text=Avoid%20fruits%20and%20vegetables%20that,or%20causing%20gas%20and%20bloating.
4. https://www.healthline.com/health/digestive-health/most-effective-diarrhea-remedies#hydration

18

Dysentery

Introduction

Dysentery is a gastrointestinal illness marked by severe diarrhoea, often accompanied by blood or mucus. There are two primary types:

1. **Amoebic Dysentery (Amoebiasis)**
   - **Cause:** Most commonly caused by Entamoeba histolytica (E. histolytica).
   - **Other Parasites:** Balantidium coli (B. coli) and Strongyloides species can also cause amoebic dysentery.

1. **Bacillary Dysentery**
   - **Cause:** Bacterial infections.
   - **Common Pathogens:** Shigella, Salmonella, Campylobacter, and Escherichia coli (E. coli).
   - **Prevalence:** Bacillary dysentery is the more common form.

Without prompt and appropriate treatment, dysentery can become life-threatening. If symptoms occur, it is essential to seek immediate medical care.

Causes

Dysentery, caused by parasitic or bacterial infections, is highly contagious. Understanding transmission routes is key to prevention.

1. **Transmission**
   - **Fecal–Oral Route:** Occurs when contaminated fecal matter enters the mouth.
   - **Common Scenarios:**
     - Poor hand hygiene during food preparation
     - Consumption of contaminated water
     - Sexual contact involving the anus
2. **Bacillary Dysentery**
   - **Cause:** Infiltration by foreign bacteria.
   - **Common Pathogens:**
     - Shigella (shigellosis)
     - Salmonella (salmonellosis)
     - Campylobacter (campylobacteriosis)
     - E. coli (various strains)
3. **Amoebic Dysentery**
   - **Cause:** Caused by ingestion of parasitic cysts, primarily E. histolytica.
4. **Contagious Nature**
   - Both forms are highly infectious. Spread commonly occurs via contaminated food and water or oral–anal contact.

Symptoms

Symptoms vary by type and severity:

Amoebic Dysentery

1. **Asymptomatic Cases:**
   - Many individuals carry the parasite without symptoms.
2. **Mild Symptoms:**
   - Diarrhoea (loose or watery stools)
   - Fever
   - Nausea and vomiting
   - Weight loss
   - Abdominal discomfort

3. **Complications (Rare):**
    - In rare cases, the parasite can spread and form abscesses in other organs (e.g., liver).

Bacillary Dysentery

1. **Characteristic Symptoms:**
    - Bloody or mucus-filled diarrhoea
    - High fever
    - Nausea and vomiting
    - Painful abdominal cramps
2. **Potential Severe Complications:**
    - Intestinal inflammation
    - Toxic megacolon (severe intestinal dilation)
    - Acute kidney injury

Foods to Avoid

To support recovery and reduce irritation:

1. **Fried and Greasy Foods**
    - Avoid foods high in fats or cooked in excessive oil.
2. **Gas-Producing Fruits and Vegetables**
    - Examples: broccoli, peppers, beans, peas, berries, prunes, chickpeas, leafy greens, and corn.
3. **Caffeine and Alcohol**
    - These may worsen dehydration and gastrointestinal irritation.
4. **Carbonated Beverages**
    - Eliminate sodas and fizzy drinks.
5. **Dairy Products**
    - Limit or avoid milk and dairy, especially if they aggravate symptoms.

Foods to Eat

Choose easily digestible, low-fibre, and soothing options:

1. **Bland Foods (BRAT Diet)**
    - **BRAT:** Bananas, white rice, applesauce, toast.
    - **Other Options:** Boiled potatoes, plain crackers, hot cereals (e.g., oatmeal, rice porridge).
    - Eat small, frequent meals to ease digestion.
2. **Probiotics**
    - **Recommended:** Yogurt, kefir (if dairy-tolerant), or non-dairy sources like fermented vegetables and soy products.
    - Consult a healthcare provider before starting probiotic supplements.
3. **Hydration**
    - **Fluids to Include:** Water, broths, coconut water, electrolyte drinks, and oral rehydration solutions (ORS).
    - Drink an extra cup of fluid after each loose stool to prevent dehydration.

Remedies

1. **Avoid Irritating Foods**
    - Limit foods that aggravate symptoms, such as:
        - High-fat and fried items (e.g., chips, pastries)
        - Artificial sweeteners
        - High-fructose products
        - Fatty meats (e.g., bacon)
        - High-fibre foods (e.g., legumes, cabbage, cauliflower)
    - Individuals with lactose intolerance should avoid dairy during recovery.

2. **Probiotic Support**
    - Probiotics may restore gut flora. A 2022 meta-analysis suggests they may improve stool frequency, consistency, and IBS-related symptoms.
    - More robust clinical trials are needed to confirm efficacy. Consult your doctor before use.
3. **Dietary Recovery Strategy**
    - Choose smaller, more frequent meals.
    - Prioritise sodium- and potassium-rich foods: broths, bananas, and boiled potatoes.
    - Include easily digestible, lower-fibre foods such as lean meats, white rice, and plain yogurt.

Hydration and Electrolyte Replenishment

- Drink water, diluted juices, ORS (e.g., Pedialyte), or sports drinks (e.g., Gatorade).
- Avoid caffeine, alcohol, carbonated drinks, and overly hot beverages.

Note: Seek immediate medical attention if symptoms persist beyond 48 hours, if there is blood in the stool, or if dehydration or severe abdominal pain occurs.

References:

1. https://my.clevelandclinic.org/health/diseases/23567-dysentery
2. https://medlineplus.gov/ency/patientinstructions/000121.htm#:~:text=Avoid%20fruits%20and%20vegetables%20that,or%20causing%20gas%20and%20bloating.
3. https://www.medicalnewstoday.com/articles/320124#foods-to-eat
4. https://www.medicalnewstoday.com/articles/324424#recovery-diet

19

Fever

Introduction

Fever, characterised by a temporary rise in body temperature, is a key component of the body's immune defense mechanism, most often triggered by infections. While fever typically causes discomfort in both children and adults, it usually poses no serious threat. However, in infants, even a slight elevation in temperature may indicate a more serious underlying infection.

Fever episodes generally resolve within a few days, and various over-the-counter (OTC) medications are available to alleviate symptoms. Treatment becomes necessary primarily when the fever causes significant discomfort, highlighting the body's natural ability to self-regulate in response to infection.

Causes

1. **Infections**
    - *Viral infections*
    - *Bacterial infections*

    Both can trigger an immune response, prompting the hypothalamus to raise the body's temperature.

2. **Heat-related conditions**
    - *Heat exhaustion*

    Overexertion or exposure to high temperatures can lead to elevated body temperature.

3. **Inflammatory conditions**

    - *Rheumatoid arthritis*

    Inflammation of the joints (synovium) can cause fever as part of the body's immune response.

4. **Underlying health issues**

    - *Malignant tumours*

    The presence of certain tumours may contribute to fever.

5. **Medications**

    - *Antibiotics*

    Some medications, including antibiotics, can raise body temperature.

6. **Treatment drugs**

    - *Medications for high blood pressure or seizures*

    Certain drugs used to treat hypertension or seizures may cause fever as a side effect.

7. **Immunisations**

    - *Vaccines*

    Vaccinations such as DTaP, pneumococcal, or COVID-19 vaccines may temporarily increase body temperature as part of the body's immune response.

Symptoms

- Fever is often accompanied by sweating, chills, headache, muscle aches, and loss of appetite.
- Irritability and general weakness are common.
- Dehydration may occur, underscoring the importance of adequate fluid intake.

Foods to Avoid

1. **High-fibre foods**
- Avoid whole grain cereals and related products.

2. **Pulses with husk**
- Refrain from consuming whole pulses or those with husk, as they may irritate the digestive system.

3. **Raw and pungent vegetables**
- Avoid vegetables such as cabbage, capsicum, turnip, radish, onion, and garlic.

4. **Fried and fatty foods**
- Eliminate items like pakoras, ladoos, bhaturas, and samosas, which can worsen symptoms.

5. **Chemical irritants**
- Avoid condiments, spices, pickles, and chutneys, which may cause digestive discomfort.

Foods to Eat

1. **Hydration**
- Drink plenty of fluids, including juices, soups, and other beverages, to stay well hydrated.

2. **Milk and dairy products**
- Include milk and milk-based drinks for nutritional support.

3. **Low-fibre foods**
- Choose refined cereals such as maida and suji, dehusked pulses, well-cooked fruits, soft vegetables, and potatoes.

4. **Mild desserts**
- Consume plain gelatin desserts and sweeteners like sugar, honey, and jams.

5. **Protein-rich foods**
- For nourishment and strength, include eggs, soft cheese, tender meats, fish, and poultry.

Remedies

1. **Stay hydrated**

- Replace fluids lost through sweating by drinking water, juices, broths, soups, sports drinks, and decaffeinated tea.

2. **Get adequate rest**

- Support your body's healing by sleeping 8–9 hours per night and limiting physical activity.

3. **Use OTC medications**

- Alleviate discomfort with medications such as acetaminophen, ibuprofen, aspirin, or naproxen. Follow dosage guidelines carefully and avoid aspirin in children.

4. **Exercise caution with herbal remedies**

- While herbal options like moringa and kudzu root may offer benefits, consult a healthcare provider—especially before giving them to children.

5. **Apply cooling techniques**

- Reduce fever safely by taking lukewarm baths, wearing light clothing, avoiding heavy blankets, and staying hydrated with cool or room-temperature fluids.

References:

1. https://www.mayoclinic.org/diseases-conditions/fever/symptoms-causes/syc-20352759
2. https://www.jaypeehealthcare.com/blog/viral-fever-what-foods-avoid-reduce-risk-illness#:~:text=FOOD%20TO%20AVOID&text=All%20raw%20%26%20strongly%20flavoured%20vegetables,%2C%20spices%2C%20pickle%2C%20chutney.
3. https://www.healthline.com/health/viral-fever-home-remedies#cooling-tips

20

Fungal Infection

Introduction

Fungal infections, or mycoses, represent a spectrum of diseases caused by various fungi, including yeasts and moulds. While these infections often manifest on the skin or nails, fungi also have the capacity to affect other regions of the body, including the oral cavity, respiratory system, and urinary tract. This wide-ranging potential underscores the need to understand and manage fungal infections as part of comprehensive healthcare.

Causes

Fungal infections are caused by yeasts, moulds, and other fungi, although only a few species are harmful to humans.

- Opportunistic infections may arise when fungi exploit weakened immune systems.
- Common causative agents include dermatophytes, which feed on keratin in hair, nails, and the outer skin without penetrating living tissue.
- *Candida albicans*, a yeast naturally present on the body, can cause itching and redness and may lead to serious infections under certain conditions.
- Environmental fungi such as *Histoplasma, Coccidioides, Blastomyces,* and *Aspergillus,* commonly found in soil or water, are also known to cause infections.

Symptoms

Symptoms vary depending on the type and location of the infection:

- **Superficial or subcutaneous infections** may cause itching, redness, soreness, rashes, discolored nails, white patches in the mouth or throat, loss of taste, or pain while eating.
- **Lung-related fungal infections** may lead to coughing (possibly with blood), fatigue, fever, shortness of breath, muscle or joint pain, headache, and night sweats.
- **Other systemic infections** may present as follows:
  - **Brain**: headache, fever, neck stiffness, nausea or vomiting, light sensitivity, confusion
  - **Eyes**: redness, pain, discharge, blurred vision, tearing, light sensitivity
  - **Intestines**: abdominal pain, nausea, vomiting
  - **Sinuses**: fever, nasal congestion, headache, one-sided facial swelling or pain

Foods to Avoid

1. Maintain a healthy diet by avoiding sugary and high-carbohydrate foods such as bread, pasta, sweets, and sugary beverages, which may encourage fungal growth.
2. Avoid canned, processed, or packaged foods, which can contain mould spores and high sodium levels—both conducive to fungal growth in moist environments.
3. Eliminate yeast-based products from your diet—such as beer, wine, and cereal—until the infection resolves.
4. Limit intake of peanuts, cashews, and certain chocolates, as they may contain natural microflora that support fungal proliferation. Reintroduce these foods only after significant improvement.

Foods to Eat

- Incorporate **yoghurt and probiotics** to introduce beneficial bacteria that help fight fungal overgrowth.
- **Cleanse the affected area** with soap and water twice daily before applying any treatment.
- **Apple cider vinegar** may be consumed in warm water or applied topically for its antifungal benefits (up to three times daily).
- **Tea tree oil**, when diluted with carrier oils like coconut or olive oil, can be applied to the infected area multiple times a day.
- **Unheated coconut oil** serves as an effective antifungal when applied topically three times daily.
- **Turmeric** provides antimicrobial and anti-inflammatory support; use as a topical paste or consume in tea or warm water.
- **Aloe vera** can soothe irritation and aid in skin repair.
- **Garlic**, mashed into a paste with olive oil, may be applied for 30 minutes daily to treat fungal skin infections.
- **Oregano oil**, either in diluted topical form or taken as capsules, offers antifungal effects.
- **Neem leaves** can be boiled to make a cleansing solution; use to rinse infected areas for their antifungal properties.

Remedies

- Consume foods rich in **vitamin C** to enhance immune response.
- For **athlete's foot**, apply baking soda to the feet and shoes to absorb moisture and prevent further infection.
- Soak feet in a 1:1 solution of water and **hydrogen peroxide** for fungal relief.

- Add **ginger** to your diet for its antifungal properties, particularly against Candida.
- Apply **honey** to affected skin for its healing and antifungal action, aided by naturally occurring hydrogen peroxide.
- Use **grapefruit seed extract** diluted in water on affected areas twice daily.
- Boil **powdered liquorice** in water, allow it to cool, and apply the paste to the skin twice daily for its anti-inflammatory and antimicrobial effects.
- Apply **lemongrass oil**, diluted with a carrier oil, using a cotton swab twice daily for its antifungal benefits.

References:

1. https://my.clevelandclinic.org/health/diseases/24401-fungal-infections-mycosis
2. https://www.secondmedic.com/app/ask/which-food-should-we-avoid-for-fungal-infection
3. https://pharmeasy.in/blog/try-these-simple-home-remedies-for-fungal-infections/#:~:text=1.-,Eat%20Yoghurt%20and%20Probiotics,another%20excellent%20source%20of%20probiotics.

21

Gallbladder Stone

Introduction

Gallstones are hardened deposits of digestive fluid—bile—that can form in the gallbladder, a small, pear-shaped organ located beneath the liver on the right side of the abdomen. This organ plays a vital role in digestion by storing bile, which is released into the small intestine when needed. Bile, produced by the liver, helps digest fats. The gallbladder contracts during meals to release bile into the small intestine, aiding the digestive process.

Gallstones vary greatly in size, from tiny particles resembling grains of sand to larger formations as big as golf balls. Some individuals may develop a single stone, while others may have multiple stones simultaneously.

When gallstones cause symptoms, surgical removal of the gallbladder is often necessary. However, asymptomatic gallstones—those causing no noticeable signs—typically do not require treatment. Understanding the formation and impact of gallstones is key to managing their potential health effects.

Causes

1. An excess of cholesterol in bile may lead to crystallisation and eventual gallstone formation.
2. Excessive bilirubin—a byproduct of red blood cell breakdown—can contribute to stone formation, particularly in conditions such as cirrhosis or blood disorders.

3. Incomplete emptying of the gallbladder can cause bile to become overly concentrated, increasing the likelihood of stone development.

Symptoms

1. Gallstones may be asymptomatic; however, if one blocks a bile duct, it can cause intense pain in the upper right abdomen.
2. Blockage may also result in sudden, severe pain in the center of the abdomen or just beneath the breastbone.
3. Pain may radiate to the back between the shoulder blades or to the right shoulder.
4. Nausea and vomiting often accompany gallstone-related pain, which can last from several minutes to a few hours.

Foods to Avoid

1. Reduce saturated and trans fats—found in whole milk, red meat, butter, ghee, cheese, cakes, biscuits, and pastries—to ease strain on the gallbladder.
2. Choose smaller, more frequent meals and replace unhealthy fats with unsaturated fats.
3. Avoid deep-fried and processed foods high in fat and sugar, as they may harm gallbladder function.
4. Choose whole grains over refined flour in products such as pasta and bread to help lower the risk of gallbladder issues.
5. Limit high-sugar foods like cakes, biscuits, and sweet baked goods to reduce the likelihood of gallstone formation.
6. Avoid rapid weight loss from extreme low-calorie diets, which can worsen symptoms and trigger gallstone formation. Instead, aim for gradual weight loss through a balanced diet and regular exercise.

7. Minimise alcohol and tobacco use, maintain a food diary to track potential triggers, and consult a general practitioner or nutritionist for personalised dietary advice.

Foods to Eat

1. Support gallbladder health by eating at least five servings of fruits and vegetables daily. Beans, citrus fruits, and leafy greens provide vitamins, minerals, fibre, and antioxidants.
2. Maintain a fibre-rich diet with fruits, vegetables, legumes, oats, and whole grains to support digestive health.
3. Stay well hydrated by drinking at least two liters of fluid daily—preferably water or herbal teas.
4. Opt for high-fibre starchy carbohydrates, such as whole grains, brown rice, and wholemeal bread.
5. Maintain calcium levels by including two to three servings of low-fat dairy products daily.
6. Choose lean protein sources such as sardines, eggs, beans, lentils, nuts, tempeh, tofu, and lean meats to support gallbladder function and reduce fat intake.
7. Replace saturated fats with healthy plant-based fats from avocados, nuts, seeds, and oils like olive, rapeseed, and sunflower oil.

Remedies

1. **Gallbladder Cleanse**: Some advocate gallbladder cleanses to dissolve stones, but no scientific evidence supports their effectiveness. Consult your doctor before trying such methods.
2. **Apple Juice**: Anecdotal claims suggest apple juice softens gallstones, though no scientific studies confirm this. Excessive juice intake may be harmful in certain conditions.
3. **Apple Cider Vinegar**: Popular in cleansing trends, apple cider vinegar has no proven benefit for gallstone treatment.

4. **Yoga**: While yoga may relieve some gallstone symptoms, there is no scientific evidence that it treats gallstones directly.
5. **Milk Thistle**: Traditionally used for liver and gallbladder health, milk thistle lacks specific research on gallstones. Consult a doctor before use.
6. **Artichoke**: Although artichoke may support gallbladder function, studies on its role in treating gallstones are lacking. It is generally safe to consume.
7. **Gold Coin Grass:** Used in traditional Chinese medicine, gold coin grass is believed to reduce gallstone formation. Seek professional guidance before use.
8. **Castor Oil Pack:** A traditional remedy said to ease gallstone pain, castor oil packs lack scientific support. Use cautiously and consult a healthcare provider.
9. **Acupuncture**: Some report pain relief from acupuncture; however, more research is needed. Ensure treatment is performed by a licensed practitioner using sterile, single-use needles.

References

1. https://www.mayoclinic.org/diseases-conditions/gallstones/symptoms-causes/syc-20354214
2. https://www.nhs.uk/conditions/gallstones/prevention/
3. https://www.spirehealthcare.com/health-hub/specialties/lifestyle-management/gallstones-diet/
4. https://www.healthline.com/health/how-to-get-rid-of-gallstones#other-treatments

22

Hair Loss

Introduction

Seeing hair everywhere can feel deeply discouraging. It may seem as though all your hair treatments are in vain and that nothing can be done.

Hair loss—medically known as alopecia—is a condition that goes beyond mere cosmetic concern. It can affect not only the scalp but also the entire body. Whether temporary or permanent, hair loss may result from a wide range of causes, including genetic predisposition, hormonal changes, underlying medical conditions, or the natural process of aging. While it affects both men and women, it is generally more prevalent in men.

The term baldness specifically refers to excessive hair loss from the scalp, commonly due to hereditary factors and aging. Some individuals embrace this natural process, while others may choose to conceal it using hairstyles, makeup, hats, or scarves.

For those seeking to prevent further hair loss or encourage regrowth, a variety of treatments are available. Addressing hair loss involves navigating a complex interplay of genetics, health, and personal choice.

Causes

1. On average, individuals naturally shed 50 to 100 hairs per day, balanced by new hair growth to maintain appearance.

2. The most common cause of hair loss is hereditary, developing gradually with age and known as androgenic alopecia (male- or female-pattern baldness).
3. Hormonal changes due to pregnancy, childbirth, menopause, or thyroid conditions can cause both temporary and permanent hair loss. Medical conditions such as alopecia areata and trichotillomania may also be contributing factors.
4. Certain medications for cancer, arthritis, depression, heart problems, and high blood pressure can lead to hair loss as a side effect.
5. Radiation therapy to the head can affect hair regrowth, potentially altering texture or density.
6. Significant physical or emotional stress can trigger temporary hair loss, which often presents as general thinning several months after the stressful event.
7. Hairstyles that exert tension—such as tight pigtails or cornrows—can lead to traction alopecia. Hair treatments like hot-oil applications and permanents may also cause hair loss, which can be permanent if scarring occurs.

Symptoms

1. Hair loss can occur suddenly or gradually and may affect the scalp or the entire body.
2. Gradual thinning on the top of the head is the most common form. Men often notice a receding hairline, while women may see a widening part or frontal fibrosing alopecia.
3. Circular or patchy bald spots may develop on the scalp, beard, or eyebrows and are sometimes preceded by itching or pain.
4. Sudden loosening of hair—often triggered by physical or emotional shock—may result in excessive hair fall during combing or washing, leading to temporary thinning.

5. Medical treatments such as chemotherapy can cause full-body hair loss; however, hair typically regrows after treatment concludes.
6. Patches of scaling on the scalp, often a sign of ringworm, may include broken hair, redness, swelling, and occasional oozing.

Foods to Avoid

1. Excessive sugar intake spikes blood glucose levels, impairing blood circulation to hair follicles and leading to dry, brittle strands.
2. Diets high in refined carbohydrates and processed foods can elevate androgen levels, contributing to hair thinning and baldness.
3. Alcohol dehydrates the hair and reduces zinc levels—both of which are vital for hair density and strength.
4. Swordfish and other mercury-rich fish can deplete zinc stores, potentially resulting in hair thinning due to zinc deficiency.
5. Greasy and oily foods stimulate sebum overproduction, which may clog hair follicles and hinder growth, leading to thinning hair.
6. Carbonated beverages containing artificial sweeteners may disrupt insulin function and blood circulation, depriving follicles of essential nutrients.

Foods to Eat

1. Eggs, rich in lutein, biotin, and vitamins A, D, and B12, are excellent sources of protein that support overall hair health.
2. Salmon, packed with omega-3 fatty acids and complete proteins, helps strengthen hair and restore its natural bounce.

3. Almond butter provides vitamin E, omega-3 and -6 fatty acids, zinc, magnesium, and iron—nutrients essential for growth and scalp health.
4. Oysters, high in zinc and omega-3s, help reduce dandruff and prevent hair loss while improving skin and scalp health.
5. Black beans, rich in lysine (an essential amino acid), promote healthy hair growth and help combat thinning.
6. Blueberries, abundant in antioxidants, enhance scalp blood flow, supporting stronger follicles and healthier hair.

Remedies

1. A Mediterranean diet rich in raw vegetables and fresh herbs—such as parsley, basil, and salad greens—may reduce the risk of androgenic alopecia when consumed at least three times a week.
2. Protein, a fundamental building block of keratin (which makes up hair), can be found in eggs, nuts, beans, fish, poultry, and low-fat dairy.
3. Vitamin A, found in foods like sweet potatoes, sweet peppers, and spinach, supports healthy hair growth—but must be consumed in moderation to prevent damage.
4. A daily multivitamin with vitamins A, B, C, and D, as well as iron, selenium, and zinc, can support cell turnover and hair retention.
5. Vitamin D deficiency is linked to nonscarring alopecia; supplementation may aid regrowth in such cases.
6. Biotin (vitamin B7 or H), essential for fatty acid synthesis, can prevent hair loss when levels are deficient.
7. Saw palmetto, derived from the American dwarf palm tree, may help balance testosterone levels and improve hair thickness and density.

8. Ginseng contains phytochemicals that may stimulate scalp hair growth, though exact dosages require further research.
9. Regular washing with a mild shampoo keeps the scalp clean and may help prevent hair loss.
10. Coconut oil, rich in lauric acid, binds to hair proteins and protects against UV damage and grooming-related breakage. Scalp massage with coconut oil may also improve blood flow.
11. Olive oil works as a deep conditioner, preventing dryness and breakage while potentially slowing genetic hair loss.
12. Gentle styling practices—such as avoiding tight hairstyles, air-drying hair, and limiting heat exposure—can help reduce breakage and scalp irritation.

References:

1. https://www.mayoclinic.org/diseases-conditions/hair-loss/symptoms-causes/syc-20372926
2. https://in.sugarcosmetics.com/blog/foods-that-cause-hair-loss
3. https://www.healthline.com/health/hair-loss-prevention#hair-care

23

Headache

Introduction

A headache is more than just pain in the head or face—it can present as a throbbing pressure, a constant ache, or a sharp or dull sensation. These discomforts vary in type, severity, location, and frequency.

Headaches are among the most commonly experienced forms of pain and are a leading cause of missed days at work or school, as well as visits to healthcare providers.

While most headaches are not dangerous, some may indicate more serious underlying conditions.

Types of Headaches

There are over 150 types of headaches, which fall into two main categories: primary and secondary.

Primary Headaches

These result from dysfunction or overactivity in pain-sensitive structures in the head and are not caused by an underlying medical condition. Examples include tension-type headaches (the most common), migraines, cluster headaches, and new daily persistent headaches.

Lifestyle factors such as alcohol consumption, specific foods, nicotine, changes in sleep, poor posture, physical activity, skipped meals, or actions like coughing or sneezing may trigger primary headaches.

Although typically not dangerous, primary headaches can be intensely painful and disruptive to daily life.

Secondary Headaches

These are caused by an underlying medical condition and act as a symptom or warning sign. Examples include dehydration headaches, sinus headaches, and medication overuse headaches.

Some secondary headaches may indicate serious or life-threatening conditions. For instance, spinal headaches (often following a spinal tap) and thunderclap headaches (sudden and intense) can point to problems such as head injury, brain bleeding, reversible cerebral vasoconstriction syndrome, or a rapid, severe rise in blood pressure.

Understanding the type of headache is crucial for appropriate management and timely medical attention—especially for secondary headaches that signal potentially serious conditions.

Causes

1. Headache pain stems from complex interactions among the brain, blood vessels, and nerves, with specific mechanisms activating pain-signaling nerves during an episode.
2. The most common cause is the activation of nerves that influence muscles and blood vessels, sending pain signals to the brain.
3. These intricate interactions can be triggered by various internal and external stimuli, including stress, dehydration, or dietary triggers.

Symptoms

1. Seek immediate medical attention if you experience a sudden, severe headache, particularly if accompanied by fever, shortness of breath, stiff neck, or rash.

2. Headaches following a head injury, or the appearance of a new headache type after age 55, or those with neurological symptoms such as weakness, dizziness, or numbness, require prompt medical evaluation.
3. Neurological symptoms such as sudden loss of balance, paralysis, speech difficulties, seizures, or vision changes also necessitate immediate attention.

Foods to Avoid

1. Migraine triggers often include foods high in tyramine, such as aged cheeses, smoked fish, and Chianti wine.
2. Red wine, caffeine (found in coffee, tea, and colas), and nitrate-rich foods like pepperoni and hot dogs are common culprits.
3. Dried fruits, potato chips, pizza, peanuts, and chicken livers may provoke migraines in some individuals.
4. Yeast-containing baked goods (e.g., sourdough bread, bagels), chocolate, cultured dairy products, and certain fruits (e.g., citrus, bananas, avocados) can act as triggers.
5. Nuts, olives, soy products (e.g., miso, tempeh, soy sauce), tomatoes, and fermented vegetables like sauerkraut may also trigger symptoms.

   Vinegar should be avoided by those sensitive to migraines.

Foods to Eat

1. Eggs, naturally rich in riboflavin (vitamin B2), may help prevent migraine headaches.
2. Watermelon, with its high water content, can help prevent dehydration—a potential headache trigger.
3. Navy beans, a magnesium-rich legume, may aid in regulating muscle function, blood sugar, and blood pressure, thereby reducing migraine frequency.

4. Almonds, rich in magnesium and vitamin E, also offer fibre, biotin, and calcium, supporting overall health and headache prevention.

Remedies

1. **Hydration:** Dehydration is a common headache trigger. Increasing water intake may reduce the occurrence, duration, and severity of headaches.
2. **Magnesium:** This essential mineral is effective in managing migraines. Start with smaller supplement doses to avoid digestive discomfort.
3. **Limit Alcohol:** Alcohol triggers migraines in about one-third of frequent headache sufferers. Reducing intake may ease symptoms.
4. **Prioritise Sleep:** Both too little and too much sleep can contribute to headaches. Aim for 7–9 hours of quality sleep nightly.
5. **Avoid Histamine-Rich Foods:** Aged cheeses and fermented products can trigger migraines in sensitive individuals. Eliminating them may help.
6. **Essential Oils:** Peppermint, lavender, and eucalyptus oils may relieve headaches. Use through diffusion or topical application.
7. **B-Complex Vitamins:** Riboflavin (B2), folate, B12, and pyridoxine (B6) may help prevent headaches. B-complex supplements are a natural option.
8. **Cold Compress:** Applying a cold compress to the head or neck may reduce inflammation and constrict blood vessels, easing pain.
9. **Coenzyme Q10 (CoQ10):** This naturally occurring substance may reduce the frequency, severity, and duration of migraines when taken as a supplement.

10. **Elimination Diet**: Identifying food intolerances by removing common triggers (e.g., aged cheeses, alcohol, chocolate, citrus fruits, coffee) may reduce headache symptoms.

References:

1. https://my.clevelandclinic.org/health/diseases/9639-headaches
2. https://www.webmd.com/migraines-headaches/avoiding-migraine-triggers
3. https://www.advil.com/symptoms-tips/pain/headache/foods-that-help-headaches/
4. https://www.healthline.com/nutrition/headache-remedies#remedies

24

Hiccups

Introduction

Hiccups—those involuntary and often amusing spasms of the diaphragm—produce a peculiar "hic" sound as the vocal cords abruptly close. This common phenomenon occurs when the diaphragm, a crucial respiratory muscle, experiences sudden, uncontrolled contractions.

While hiccups are typically short-lived—often triggered by overeating, drinking alcoholic or carbonated beverages, or experiencing sudden excitement—persistent or prolonged hiccups can indicate an underlying medical concern. Although most episodes resolve within minutes, in rare cases, hiccups that persist for weeks or even months may lead to weight loss and significant fatigue. In such cases, medical evaluation is warranted to identify potential causes.

Causes

1. Short-term hiccups (lasting less than 48 hours) can be triggered by:
   - Drinking carbonated beverages
   - Excessive alcohol consumption
   - Overeating
   - Emotional stress
   - Sudden temperature changes
   - Activities like chewing gum or smoking

2. Persistent hiccups (lasting more than 48 hours) may result from:
    - Nerve damage or irritation (particularly to the phrenic or vagus nerves)
    - Central nervous system disorders such as stroke, encephalitis, or multiple sclerosis
    - Metabolic conditions like diabetes or kidney failure
    - Reactions to certain medications or substances, including alcohol or anaesthesia

Symptoms

The hallmark symptom of hiccups is an involuntary contraction of the diaphragm, followed by a quick closure of the vocal cords, producing the characteristic "hic" sound. In addition to this audible reflex, individuals may experience a subtle tightening sensation in the chest, abdomen, or throat. These physical cues accompany the spasmodic activity and signal the presence of ongoing diaphragm irritation.

Foods to Avoid

To help prevent or reduce hiccup episodes, it is advisable to avoid:

1. Overeating or eating too quickly
2. Spicy or extremely hot foods
3. Alcoholic beverages
4. Carbonated drinks
5. Sudden temperature changes in food or drink (e.g., hot soup followed by cold water)

Some cultural beliefs associate hiccups with superstitions (e.g., "someone is thinking of you"), but these should not replace a physiological understanding of the condition.

Foods to Eat

While scientific evidence is limited, certain foods are traditionally used as natural remedies to stop hiccups by stimulating the vagus nerve or distracting the body's reflexive patterns:

1. **Honey**: Soothes the vagus nerve, interrupting the hiccup reflex
2. **Vinegar**: Its sharp taste may distract the nervous system and reset diaphragm control
3. **Sugar**: A spoonful of granulated sugar may irritate the oesophagus just enough to disrupt the reflex arc
4. **Peanut butter**: Its thick texture alters breathing and swallowing patterns, possibly resetting the diaphragm
5. **Lemon**: Its high acidity and sharp taste can distract the vagus nerve; sucking on a lemon wedge may help

Remedies

Several simple home remedies aim to interrupt the reflex cycle and relax the diaphragm:

1. **Measured breathing**: Inhale for a count of five, then exhale for a count of five
2. **Breath-holding**: Take a deep breath and hold it for 10 to 20 seconds
3. **Paper bag breathing**: Slowly inhale and exhale into a paper (not plastic) bag to increase carbon dioxide levels, which may relax the diaphragm
4. **Knee-to-chest position**: While seated, hug your knees to your chest to apply pressure on the diaphragm
5. **Valsalva manoeuvre**: Exhale forcefully while pinching your nose and keeping your mouth closed
6. **Tongue pull**: Gently pull on your tongue to stimulate the throat and diaphragm muscles

7. **Nasal and neck stimulation**: Lightly squeeze the nose or massage the carotid artery area (with caution) to stimulate the vagus nerve

References:

1. https://timesofindia.indiatimes.com/life-style/food-news/these-6-foods-can-give-immediate-relief-from-hiccups/photostory/71971608.cms?picid=71971627
2. https://www.mayoclinic.org/diseases-conditions/hiccups/symptoms-causes/syc-20352613
3. https://www.healthline.com/health/how-to-get-rid-of-hiccups#when-to-see-a-doctor

25

High Blood Pressure

Introduction

High blood pressure, also known as **hypertension**, is a prevalent condition that affects the arteries of the body. It occurs when the force exerted by the blood against the arterial walls remains consistently elevated. As a result, the heart must work harder to pump blood throughout the circulatory system.

Blood pressure is measured in millimetres of mercury (mm Hg), with hypertension typically identified by a reading of **130/80 mm Hg or higher**. The American College of Cardiology and the American Heart Association classify blood pressure according to the following categories:

1. **Normal blood pressure**: 120/80 mm Hg or lower
2. **Elevated blood pressure**: Systolic (top number) between 120 and 129 mm Hg, and diastolic (bottom number) below 80 mm Hg
3. **Stage 1 hypertension**: Systolic between 130 and 139 mm Hg or diastolic between 80 and 89 mm Hg
4. **Stage 2 hypertension**: Systolic of 140 mm Hg or higher or diastolic of 90 mm Hg or higher

A blood pressure reading exceeding **180/120 mm Hg** constitutes a **hypertensive emergency** and requires immediate medical attention. Left untreated, high blood pressure significantly increases the risk of heart attacks, strokes, and other serious health complications. Routine blood pressure monitoring–ideally every two years beginning at age

18—is essential. Adopting a healthy lifestyle, including regular exercise, a balanced diet, and the avoidance of tobacco, is key to prevention and management. In some cases, medication may also be required.

Causes

1. **Blood pressure basics:** Blood pressure depends on how much blood the heart pumps and the resistance in the arteries; increased pumping or narrower arteries lead to higher pressure.
2. **Primary hypertension:** Often develops gradually over several years without a specific cause (also called essential hypertension). Atherosclerosis is a contributing risk factor.
3. **Secondary hypertension:** Arises suddenly and tends to cause higher readings than primary hypertension. It is caused by underlying health issues, such as kidney disease, thyroid dysfunction, or certain medications.
4. **Triggers of secondary hypertension:** Include adrenal gland tumours, congenital heart defects, certain drugs, illegal substances, and obstructive sleep apnoea.
5. **White coat hypertension:** Elevated blood pressure observed during medical visits but not reflective of normal daily levels.

Symptoms

1. **The silent presence:** Hypertension typically produces no symptoms—even at dangerously high levels—making it a "silent killer" that may go undetected for years.
2. **Rare symptoms:** In some cases, individuals may experience headaches, shortness of breath, or nosebleeds. However, these symptoms are nonspecific and usually occur only in severe or prolonged hypertension.

Foods to Avoid

1. **Salt awareness:** Reducing sodium intake is crucial for managing high blood pressure. Hidden sources include sauces, canned goods, packaged snacks, and processed meats.
2. **Sugar moderation:** Excess sugar contributes to hypertension and weight gain. Limit sweets, carbonated drinks, and high-sugar packaged products.
3. **Fat consciousness:** Avoid unhealthy fats found in fried foods and highly processed items. Choose low-fat or skimmed dairy alternatives.
4. **Alcohol caution:** Limit or abstain from alcohol. If consuming, do so moderately—ideally, one drink per occasion and only occasionally.

Foods to Eat

1. **Vegetables and fruits boost:** Incorporate more vitamin-rich produce with a low glycaemic index to support heart health and regulate blood pressure.
2. **Whole grain goodness:** Choose whole grains such as oats, quinoa, and brown rice over refined flour products for sustained energy and fibre.
3. **Protein picks:** Opt for lean protein sources, including fish, skinless poultry, and plant-based options like legumes, nuts, and seeds.

Remedies

1. **Get moving for heart health:** Engage in regular physical activity. Exercise not only lowers blood pressure but also improves mood, strength, and balance. Outdoor activities like walking, swimming, or cycling are excellent choices.

2. **DASH your way to lower blood pressure**: The **DASH diet** (Dietary Approaches to Stop Hypertension) emphasises fruits, vegetables, whole grains, lean proteins, and minimal saturated fats, significantly reducing systolic pressure.
3. **Sodium scrutiny**: Aim to keep sodium intake between **1,500 and 2,300 mg per day.** Use herbs and spices instead of salt, and avoid processed foods with hidden sodium.
4. **Weight matters:** Losing just **5 to 10 pounds (2.2 to 4.5 kg)** can significantly reduce blood pressure, especially in individuals who are overweight. Maintain a healthy waist circumference: under 40 inches (102 cm) for men and 35 inches (89 cm) for women.
5. **Quit smoking for a healthy heart**: Smoking temporarily increases blood pressure and poses long-term cardiovascular risks. Quitting improves overall heart health and reduces stroke risk.
6. **Moderate alcohol intake**: While moderate consumption—especially red wine—may have some cardiovascular benefits, excessive drinking raises blood pressure. Follow AHA guidelines: up to **two drinks per day for men** and **one for women**.
7. **Stress less for lower pressure**: Identify and manage chronic stressors. Relaxation techniques such as deep breathing, meditation, and yoga may help reduce blood pressure and enhance well-being.

References:

1. https://www.mayoclinic.org/diseases-conditions/high-blood-pressure/symptoms-causes/syc-20373410
2. https://pharmeasy.in/blog/4-foods-to-avoid-if-you-have-high-bp/
3. https://www.healthline.com/health/high-blood-pressure-home-remedies#reduce-stress

26

Hair Psoriasis

Introduction

Hair psoriasis, scientifically known as scalp psoriasis, is a persistent autoimmune condition in which the immune system triggers rapid skin cell reproduction. This results in the formation of thick, discolored patches called plaques. These plaques commonly appear on the scalp and surrounding areas, including the hairline, forehead, back of the neck, and around the ears. Understanding scalp psoriasis requires recognizing its chronic nature and the impact it has on skin health in these regions.

Causes

1. Scalp psoriasis results from an overactive immune system, which leads to inflammation and the rapid growth of new skin cells.
2. Unlike the normal skin cell cycle of twenty-eight to thirty days, individuals with scalp psoriasis experience new cell growth every three to four days, leading to thick patches of skin.
3. Although there is a genetic component—scalp psoriasis often runs in families—various triggers can contribute to flare-ups. These include environmental factors such as skin trauma, sunburn, medications, stress, and other inflammatory or autoimmune conditions.

Symptoms

1. **Mild symptoms:** Characterised by small, thin scales or dandruff-like flaking.

2. **Moderate to severe symptoms:**

    - Raised, discolored plaques covered with white or silvery dead skin cells
    - Plaques that may cover most or all of the scalp
    - Involvement of the hairline, forehead, back of the neck, and areas around the ears
    - Additional symptoms: dryness, flaking, itching, fissures (cracks), bleeding, irritation, and pain

Symptoms can range from mild discomfort to severe, visibly distressing conditions that affect overall scalp health and quality of life.

Foods to Avoid

1. **Junk Foods and Inflammation**

    - High in unhealthy fats and sugars, junk foods promote inflammation and are best avoided.

    - These foods also contribute to weight gain, which is common among people with psoriasis.

2. **Red Meats and Arachidonic Acid**

    - Red meats contain arachidonic acid, a polyunsaturated fat that may worsen psoriasis symptoms.

    - Processed meats such as sausage and bacon should also be avoided.

3. **Nightshade Vegetables**

    - Some individuals experience flare-ups after consuming vegetables in the nightshade family, such as peppers, white potatoes, eggplant, and tomatoes.

    - These contain solanine, a compound that may trigger pain or inflammation in sensitive individuals.

4. **Allergenic Citrus Fruits**
    - Citrus fruits such as grapefruit, oranges, lemons, and limes may trigger allergic reactions and exacerbate psoriasis symptoms.
5. **Gluten and Grains**
    - Avoiding gluten-containing grains (wheat, rye, and barley) may help reduce symptoms, particularly for those with gluten sensitivity.
6. **Certain Condiments and Spices**
    - Condiments and spices including pimento, cinnamon, curry, vinegar, mayonnaise, paprika, Tabasco sauce, Worcestershire sauce, and ketchup may trigger inflammation in some people with psoriasis.

Foods to Eat

1. **Anti-Inflammatory Foods**
    - A whole-food, anti-inflammatory diet may reduce the frequency and severity of psoriasis flare-ups.
    - The Mediterranean diet, in particular, helps combat chronic inflammation.
2. **Psoriasis-Friendly Choices**
    - Recommended foods include fish, lean or plant-based proteins (such as tofu and tempeh), fruits, vegetables, legumes, nuts, seeds, olive oil, small portions of low-fat dairy, and whole grains.
3. **Diet over Supplements**
    - There is no conclusive evidence that supplements or vitamins significantly improve psoriasis symptoms.
    - A well-rounded diet is the best source of essential nutrients. A daily multivitamin may be safe but should be discussed with your doctor or a registered dietitian.

Remedies

1. **Aloe Vera**
    - Creams containing 0.5% aloe vera may help reduce itching, inflammation, and redness.
    - Apply up to three times daily; improvements may be seen within a month.
2. **Baking Soda Solution**
    - A mixture of baking soda and water can relieve itching when applied to the scalp.
    - Pour directly onto the scalp to soothe irritation.
3. **Capsaicin (from Chili Peppers)**
    - Creams containing capsaicin may reduce pain, redness, flaking, and inflammation.
    - Use with caution—it may sting. Avoid open wounds or sensitive areas.
4. **Coconut or Avocado Oil**
    - Rich in healthy fats, these oils can moisturise and reduce scalp scaling.
    - Apply to the scalp, cover with a shower cap for 20 minutes, then wash as usual.
5. **Garlic and Aloe Vera**
    - Garlic's anti-inflammatory properties may help reduce symptoms.
    - Mix crushed garlic with aloe vera gel, apply to the scalp, and rinse after 15 to 20 minutes.
6. **Mahonia Aquifolium**
    - Creams containing 10% Mahonia aquifolium extract may reduce inflammation and other symptoms of scalp psoriasis.

7. **Oatmeal Baths**
    - Adding raw ground oats to warm bathwater may relieve itching, inflammation, and flaking.
    - Soak the affected area for best results.
8. **Omega-3 Fatty Acids**
    - Fish oil and plant-based omega-3 supplements may help reduce systemic inflammation.
    - Though not proven to target scalp psoriasis directly, they are generally safe for daily use.
9. **Sea Salt or Epsom Salt Soaks**
    - Soaking in a warm bath with dissolved sea salt or Epsom salts may ease symptoms.
    - Soak for about 15 minutes, then apply a moisturiser.
10. **Medicated Shampoos**
    - Over-the-counter shampoos containing coal tar or 2–10% salicylic acid are effective treatments.
11. **Tea Tree Oil**
    - With antiseptic properties, tea tree oil may reduce inflammation and redness.
    - However, it can cause allergic reactions or hormonal effects in some individuals—use cautiously.
12. **Turmeric**
    - Daily turmeric intake (1.5 to 3 grams) or use in cooking may help reduce symptoms.
    - Known for its anti-inflammatory effects, turmeric is generally considered safe at these doses.
13. **Sunshine and Vitamin D**
    - Sun exposure may reduce symptoms. Always wear sunscreen, and consult your doctor if you are taking medications that increase sun sensitivity.

References:

1. https://my.clevelandclinic.org/health/diseases/22828-scalp-psoriasis
2. https://www.lybrate.com/topic/scalp-psoriasis-diet
3. https://www.hopkinsmedicine.org/health/conditions-and-diseases/psoriasis-diet-foods-to-eat-and-avoid-if-you-have-psoriasis
4. https://www.healthline.com/health/scalp-psoriasis-home-remedies#home-remedies

27

Insomnia

Introduction

Insomnia is more than just a night of tossing and turning–it refers to inadequate sleep quality or quantity. This may involve difficulty falling asleep, frequent nighttime awakenings, or waking too early. For some, insomnia is a minor inconvenience; for others, it can severely disrupt daily functioning. The causes of insomnia are diverse and not yet fully understood. However, what is clear is that the body needs sufficient sleep to function optimally. Scientific research continues to uncover the critical role of sleep, and the consequences of its absence can be far-reaching and unpleasant.

Causes

1. **Multifactorial Origins**: Insomnia is a complex condition with multiple contributing factors, many of which require further research.
2. **Genetic Links**: Family history may play a role, as sleep traits and disorders often run in families.
3. **Brain Chemistry**: Differences in brain activity or neurotransmitter levels may influence sleep regulation.
4. **Medical Conditions**: Both acute and chronic illnesses, particularly those affecting the circadian rhythm, can impair sleep.
5. **Mental Health Disorders**: Anxiety, depression, and other psychiatric conditions frequently coexist with chronic insomnia.

6. **Stressful Circumstances**: High-stress life events may contribute to insomnia, even if they are not the sole cause.
7. **Life Changes**: Temporary or long-term disruptions—such as jet lag or moving homes—can disturb sleep patterns.
8. **Sleep Hygiene**: Poor habits, including irregular sleep schedules, excessive napping, and high caffeine intake, can lead to insomnia.

Symptoms

1. **Varied Manifestations:** Insomnia symptoms are typically grouped into sleep disturbances, daytime consequences, and chronic indicators.
2. **Sleep Difficulties:** These may include:
    - *Initial insomnia*: difficulty falling asleep.
    - *Middle insomnia*: waking during the night.
    - *Late insomnia*: waking too early and being unable to return to sleep.
3. **Daytime Impacts:** These include fatigue, delayed reaction times, memory issues, slowed thinking, mood disturbances, and difficulty performing daily tasks.
4. **Chronic Insomnia**: Defined by symptoms occurring at least three times per week for at least three months, without a clear explanation such as medication use or other sleep disorders.

Foods to Avoid

1. **Caffeine**: Found in coffee, soda, energy drinks, and chocolate, caffeine is a stimulant that can delay sleep onset and impair sleep quality.
2. **Spicy Foods**: These can cause indigestion or acid reflux, particularly at night, and may elevate body temperature, interfering with sleep.

3. **Sugary and High-Glycemic Foods:** Foods high in refined carbohydrates and sugars can cause blood sugar fluctuations that negatively affect hormone balance and sleep quality.
4. **Fatty Foods:** Diets high in saturated and trans fats may lead to less restorative sleep. Heavy meals close to bedtime can strain digestion and contribute to reflux or discomfort.

Foods to Eat

Certain foods are associated with improved sleep due to their nutritional profiles. However, nutrient content can vary widely depending on variety, climate, and cultivation practices.

1. **Kiwi**
    - Rich in vitamins C and E, potassium, and folate.
    - Eating two kiwis before bed may improve sleep duration and quality, potentially due to serotonin and antioxidant effects.
2. **Tart Cherries**
    - Contain more melatonin than sweet cherries.
    - Tart cherry juice has been shown to increase sleep duration and efficiency.
3. **Malted Milk**
    - A mixture of milk and malted grain powder.
    - May reduce nighttime awakenings, possibly due to vitamins B and D.
    - Night-milked cows' milk may contain more melatonin.
4. **Fatty Fish**
    - Fish such as salmon, when consumed three times per week, may enhance sleep quality and daytime alertness.
    - Benefits are attributed to vitamin D and omega-3 fatty acids.

5. **Nuts**
    - Almonds, walnuts, pistachios, and cashews contain melatonin, magnesium, and zinc.
    - Clinical trials suggest that these nutrients support sleep, especially in older adults with insomnia.
6. **Rice**
    - High-glycemic-index rice may improve sleep, potentially due to its effect on tryptophan absorption when paired with moderate protein intake.

Remedies

1. **Progressive Muscle Relaxation (PMR)**
    - A stress-reducing technique involving the systematic tensing and relaxing of muscle groups.
    - Recommended by the American Academy of Sleep Medicine for managing chronic insomnia.
2. **Magnesium**
    - Supports muscle relaxation and stress reduction.
    - Daily supplementation or consumption of magnesium-rich foods (e.g., bananas, leafy greens, warm milk) may enhance sleep quality and duration.
3. **Regular Exercise**
    - Engaging in at least 150 minutes of physical activity per week improves sleep, mood, and overall health.
    - Low-impact activities such as walking, swimming, or yoga, especially earlier in the day, are particularly beneficial.
4. **Good Sleep Hygiene**
    - Practices include a consistent sleep schedule, limited screen time before bed, and creating a restful bedroom environment.

- Avoiding stimulating activities in the evening can further improve sleep quality.

5. **Lavender Oil**
   - Used in aromatherapy to promote relaxation.
   - Lavender diffusers or patches, when combined with good sleep hygiene, may improve sleep onset and quality.
6. **Valerian Root**
   - A herbal remedy available in tea, tincture, capsule, or tablet form.
   - May improve sleep when taken in doses ranging from 400 to 900 mg before bedtime.
   - Consultation with a healthcare provider or qualified herbalist is advised.
7. **Chamomile**
   - Known for its calming effects and typically consumed as a tea or supplement.
   - May improve sleep quality, particularly in older adults.
8. **Mindful Meditation**
   - Reduces stress and improves overall well-being.
   - Studies suggest it helps decrease total wake time and supports sleep.
   - Mindfulness practices are available through mobile apps, online videos, in-person classes, and retreats.

These lifestyle adjustments and natural remedies may help manage insomnia and promote restful sleep. However, individuals with persistent or severe symptoms should consult a medical professional for comprehensive evaluation and care.

References:

1. https://my.clevelandclinic.org/health/diseases/12119-insomnia
2. https://www.healthline.com/nutrition/foods-that-keep-you-awake#4.-Fatty-foods
3. https://www.sleepfoundation.org/nutrition/food-and-drink-promote-good-nights-sleep#:~:text=Foods%20like%20kiwi%2C%20cherries%2C%20milk,for%20maintaining%20healthy%20sleep%20patterns.
4. https://www.medicalnewstoday.com/articles/home-remedies-for-insomnia#pmr

28

Intestinal Parasites

Introduction

Intestinal parasites, commonly known as intestinal worms, are a significant category of parasites that affect the human digestive system. While these parasites are especially prevalent in subtropical and tropical regions, certain types are also found in the United States. Despite their geographical spread, most infections typically result in mild illnesses and can be effectively managed with appropriate medication. This section explores the nature, causes, symptoms, and treatments of intestinal worm infections.

Causes

1. **Undercooked Meat**: Consuming undercooked meat—especially from infected animals such as cows, pigs, or fish—can lead to intestinal worm infections. These meats may harbour live parasites that enter the digestive system and cause infection.
2. **Contaminated Water or Soil**: Drinking contaminated water or ingesting soil containing parasite eggs or larvae can introduce parasites into the digestive tract, resulting in infection.
3. **Contact with Contaminated Feces**: Exposure to feces containing parasite eggs or larvae, often due to poor hygiene or environmental conditions, can transmit intestinal worms.

4. **Poor Sanitation and Hygiene**: Inadequate sanitation and hygiene increase the risk of exposure to contaminated materials, thereby facilitating parasite transmission.
5. **Lifecycle and Infection Process**: After ingestion, parasites travel to the intestines, where they reproduce and grow. The resulting increase in parasite numbers and size typically leads to the onset of symptoms.

Symptoms

1. Abdominal pain, diarrhea, nausea, vomiting, gas, bloating, fatigue, and unexplained weight loss
2. Dysentery, characterised by diarrhea with blood and mucus in the stool
3. Rash or itching around the rectum or vulva
4. Passage of a visible worm in the stool
5. Asymptomatic cases, where the individual carries worms for extended periods without noticeable symptoms

Foods to Avoid

1. **Sugar and Simple Carbohydrates**: Parasites thrive on glucose. Avoid refined carbohydrates such as bread, pasta, rice, and sugary fruits like mangoes and grapes. When uncertain, consult a healthcare provider.
2. **Coffee, Meat, and Dairy**: These foods create an acidic internal environment that supports parasite survival. Consider limiting or avoiding these during a cleanse.
3. **Alcohol**: Since both alcohol and medications like metronidazole are processed by the liver, consuming alcohol during or shortly after treatment may increase liver toxicity. Avoid it to reduce strain on the liver.

Foods to Eat

1. **Garlic:** Chewing or chopping garlic activates allicin, a compound with antiparasitic properties. It can be consumed raw or in capsule form, though raw garlic may be more effective.
2. **Papaya Seeds:** Consuming papaya seeds on an empty stomach can help eliminate parasites. Their strong taste can be masked in a smoothie. Begin with a small quantity and gradually increase to avoid side effects.
3. **Coconut Oil:** Rich in saturated fats, coconut oil transforms into compounds that may kill harmful organisms. Incorporating it into meals may offer therapeutic benefits.
4. **Oil of Oregano:** Oregano oil is known for its antiparasitic, antiviral, antibacterial, and antifungal properties. Rich in antioxidants, it may aid in treating parasitic infections.

Remedies and Preventive Measures

1. **Handwashing:** Wash hands thoroughly with soap and hot water before and after using the toilet and before preparing or consuming food to reduce the risk of ingesting parasites.
2. **Avoid Raw Meat and Fish:** Raw meats can harbour parasites. Ensure thorough cooking to kill harmful organisms.
3. **Cooking Temperatures:** Cook meats to a minimum of 145°F (62.8°C) for whole cuts and 160°F (71°C) for ground meat and poultry. Let meat rest for three minutes before cutting or serving to complete the cooking process.
4. **Freezing Meat and Fish:** Freeze at -4°F (-20°C) for at least 24 hours to kill parasites.
5. **Wash, Peel, or Cook Fruits and Vegetables:** Proper handling of raw produce reduces the risk of parasite transmission.

6. **Dropped Food**: Wash or reheat any food that has come into contact with the floor to prevent contamination.

References

1. https://www.healthline.com/health/intestinal-worms#prevention
2. https://www.projectmurray.xyz/blog/advise-amoebas

Other books by Author

1. **Vitamins & Minerals**: Unlock vibrant health with the essential guide to vitamins and minerals! Explore their benefits, rich food sources, daily recommendations, and expert insights on managing deficiencies and avoiding excesses.

2. **Arthritis is Reversible**: Shatter the Myths, Embrace Hope: Your Guide to a Brighter Future with Reversible Arthritis. Unmask the misconceptions and discover natural solutions for managing and potentially reversing arthritis.

3. **Detox Your Body** (free E-book, available on author's website): Unveil your body's natural potential! Detox to eliminate toxins, discover the signs and benefits and explore a range of safe and effective methods for lasting transformation. Embrace a vibrant you. Learn why detox matters, identify the need, unlock amazing benefits, and delve into practical internal cleansing and revitalisation strategies.

4. **Decoding Obesity**: Conquer obesity! Dr. Trehan's book unveils the truth, busts myths, and empowers you. Get expert advice on food, habits, and overall health. Unlock a healthier, happier you!

5. **Knocking Depression with food**: The book links nutrition to mental health, especially depression. It explains how neurotransmitters, inflammation, and phytonutrients affect the brain, offering practical ways to include these nutrients in daily diets. It promotes a holistic approach—combining diet, exercise, stress management, and medical care—while encouraging hope and empowerment.

6. **Irresistible Detox Elixirs**: A Love Affair with Healthful Drinks: Discover rejuvenation through vibrant, nutrient-rich smoothies. These flavourful recipes cleanse, nourish, and energise—helping you feel revitalised and radiant in a hectic world.

Forthcoming Titles

1. Decoding Diabetes-Exploring the Real Cause
2. Decoding Diabetes-The Path to Reversal
3. Optimizing the Body's Repair Time: Harnessing the Power of Healing
4. Fuel Your Life: The Ultimate Guide to Optimal Health and Vitality

www.ingramcontent.com/pod-product-compliance
Ingram Content Group UK Ltd.
Pitfield, Milton Keynes, MK11 3LW, UK
UKHW021339190726
13845UKWH00027B/635

9 789334 440751